LIVER AND KIDNEY RESCUE MASTERY 2 IN 1 VALUE COLLECTION: LIVER DETOX CLEANSE + THE CELERY JUICE CLEANSE

Detox Fix for Thyroid, Weight Issues, Gout, Acne, Eczema, Psoriasis, Diabetes and Acid Reflux

GABRIELLE TOWNSEND

Silk Publishing

Gabrielle Townsend

© **Copyright 2020 / 2021 - All rights reserved.**

The content contained within this book may not be reproduced, duplicated or transmitted without direct written permission from the author or the publisher.

Under no circumstances will any blame or legal responsibility be held against the publisher, or author, for any damages, reparation, or monetary loss due to the information contained within this book, either directly or indirectly.

Legal Notice:

This book is copyright protected. It is only for personal use. You cannot amend, distribute, sell, use, quote or paraphrase any part, or the content within this book, without the consent of the author or publisher.

Disclaimer Notice:

Please note the information contained within this document is for educational and entertainment purposes only. All effort has been executed to present accurate, up to date, reliable, complete information. No warranties of any kind are declared or implied. Readers acknowledge that the author is not engaged in the rendering of legal, financial, medical or professional advice. The content within this book has been derived from various sources. Please consult a licensed professional before attempting any techniques outlined in this book.

By reading this document, the reader agrees that under no circumstances is the author responsible for any losses, direct or indirect, that are incurred as a result of the use of the information contained within this document, including, but not limited to, errors, omissions, or inaccuracies.

LIVER DETOX CLEANSE:

The Ultimate Cleansing Program *for* Long Term Liver Health

Detox Fix for Weight Issues, Gout, Acne, Eczema, SIBO & Autoimmune Disease, Adrenal Stress, Psoriasis, Diabetes, Gallstones, Strep, Bloating, Fatigue and Fatty Liver

GABRIELLE TOWNSEND

INTRODUCTION

"My body is like a temple in Nepal. It is sacred, but has a lot of damage from the earthquake of my youth!"

— JAMES HAUENSTEIN

The liver is one of the most unsung organs in the body. Normally, it goes unnoticed, helping us function without us ever realizing it. While there are cases when the liver becomes a medical focus, such as in chronic alcoholism with the threat of cirrhosis or hepatitis A, B, and C, it tends to fly under the radar, often forgotten. What most individuals don't realize is that the liver is a cleansing organ for the body that is also vital to immune system strength and health.

Before getting too deep into liver cleanses and what this book can do for you, let's talk about the liver. Out of all the solid organs in the body, the liver is one of the largest. Its primary function is to remove waste from the body. It is a natural filtration system for the body, turning toxins into waste that can be eliminated harmlessly. The liver cleanses your blood and serves as a metabolic agent in processing nutrients and medication. This process also provides the body with some very important proteins.

The liver is essential to life, and a healthy liver is essential to a healthy body. Your liver helps to regulate some important bodily functions. As such, overindulging in activities or substances that can hurt the liver will hinder those functions that are vital to keeping the body running. This information in itself is not novel or controversial. However, when it comes to keeping the liver healthy or health care providers discussing liver health as a part of everyday health, it is usually put on the back burner.

Consider how important the liver is as a natural filtration organ in the body. If that filtration system is clogged or overtaxed, toxins and harmful waste can begin to build up in the body. Those buildups can lead to conditions that appear to be unrelated to the liver, such as acne, eczema, autoimmune disorders, and adrenal stress. The best thing that you can do for your liver is to allow it to cleanse itself so that it can continue to filter your body and perform those vital functions.

The body builds up toxic junk over time. Easy access to junk food, jobs that require long hours or stationary sitting, and other commonplace occurrences in today's society slowly wear the body down. Those are the kinds of factors that begin to take a toll on the liver over years and years.

What's to be done about it? Fortunately, there are many holistic and natural approaches to improving liver health in the long term. Generally speaking, it is almost never too late to begin living healthier. Unfortunately, a lot of people in today's society don't realize they need to live healthier until they are forced to do so. That often comes with a major health crisis, scare, or life-threatening event. One of the best policies for long-term health, including liver health, is to strive toward prevention.

INTRODUCTION

Think about this: If you own a dog, your vet probably encourages you to give your dog monthly heartworm prevention pills. While it might seem expensive and excessive to give your dog a monthly treatment for something they may never get, consider what a dog goes through for heartworm treatment. A dog that has heartworm is treated with a very potent medication to flush the heartworm out of their system. If it goes untreated, the dog won't survive. The medication is so potent, though, that the treatment can result in the untimely passing of the dog as well.

This treatment is dangerous, costly, and sometimes doesn't get all the worms, so the dog has to go for another round. By giving your dog monthly heartworm preventatives, you spare them the dangerous treatment and your wallet the financial blow. Isn't that what prevention is all about, taking action in the present to avoid something worse in the future?

Another example of preventative measures is car insurance. Most drivers don't leave their driveway with the expectation of getting into a car crash. However, most drivers carry auto insurance in the event they do get into a crash. It covers medical expenses and car damages and supplies additional benefits in the unfortunate event of a car crash.

Your liver is like a dog or a car. You want to have preventative measures in place so that you can avoid liver-related problems in the future. More than that, if your liver is already overtaxed and you are experiencing the side effects of that, a liver detox and cleanse will help clear it out and let you move toward a healthier body, clearing up some long-term or chronic conditions.

By choosing to read *Liver Detox Cleanse: The Ultimate Cleansing Program for Long-Term Liver Health*, you are preparing yourself to learn a multitude of steps and lifestyle alterations that will ensure long-term liver health for you and your family.

INTRODUCTION

Please keep in mind that the information in this book is not a substitute for medical care or the diagnoses, examinations, or treatments of a qualified medical professional.

Through the course of reading this book, you will learn about your liver and why it is vital to a healthy body and life. You will also discover many techniques and methods for changing your lifestyle to maintain a healthy liver on a long-term basis. It is time to become a healthier you.

1
KNOW YOUR LIVER

Before you can understand what it is that a liver detox can do for you, you'll want a better understanding of what your liver is and why it is vital to your survival and health. This first chapter will cover everything you need to know about the liver and its function and how to know if a liver detox is right for you.

Please remember that all vital organs in your body should be cared for in ways specific to their functionality. The purpose of this book is to discuss the liver specifically and how a liver detox and lifestyle changes can improve your overall health in relation to your liver. If you have concerns about the other organs in your body, you might find that starting with your liver helps to clear up some of the issues that have led you to be concerned about the other organs.

With that in mind, let's get right into the liver!

INTRODUCTION TO THE LIVER

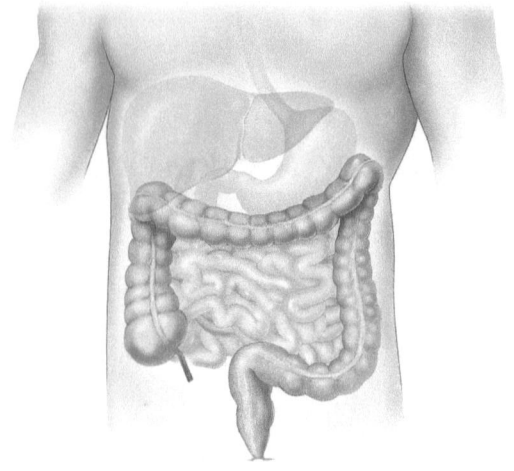

Making up roughly 2% of an adult's body weight, the liver is the largest internal human organ. The liver sits on the right side of the abdominopelvic body cavity, above the small and large intestine, slightly overlapping the stomach. The liver is vital because it supports many body systems, including the immune system, digestive system, and other metabolic processes. In fact, the liver has a role in almost every organ system within the body, such as the endocrine system and the gastrointestinal systems.

In general, the liver is responsible for keeping the blood clean, removing toxins from the blood, metabolizing sex hormones and other metabolic functions, and producing carrier proteins that contribute to reproduction and development. The liver isn't just a filtration organ, though. It also stores important minerals and vitamins, like iron and copper. It also plays an important role in cholesterol regulation.

The liver is a unique organ in that it has incredible regenerative properties. If someone needs a liver transplant, sometimes, they can get a living donor transplant. What this means is that a matching donor can donate a lobe of their liver to the patient in need of a transplant. After the lobe is properly implanted into the patient and their old liver is removed, the lobe can grow to a full, functioning size in only a few weeks. The donor doesn't lose the functionality of their liver either as the organ regenerates the lobe that was removed.

Knowing about the liver's regenerative properties makes it possible to understand that an overtaxed liver or a partially damaged liver has the potential to heal and regenerate itself if given the opportunity.

THE LIVER'S PRIMARY FUNCTION

As you may have discerned from the previous section, the liver has a lot of different functions within the body. This section is going to break down the vast array of functions into the basic functions of the liver and their importance. Having a better understanding of what your liver does inside your body will hopefully help you to see why the liver needs to be taken care of.

Bile Production

The kidneys are a waste elimination organ within the body. However, not all wastes can be eliminated by the kidneys. This is where bile comes in. One of the bile's primary functions is to excrete material that isn't eliminated through the kidneys. Bile also plays an important role in the absorption of lipids in the body. Bile is an important substance when it comes to eliminating waste in the body and also maintaining gut, intestine, and bowel health.

The liver is the organ that produces this vital bodily

substance. Bile isn't just created in the liver; it is also recycled back to the liver. Through this production and recycle system, the liver helps to create a substance the body needs and then eliminates the waste once it is used. It makes a closed system, but that system has to be kept healthy to work.

If the intestine and bowel aren't at optimal health, the body can begin to experience a lot of issues, including irritable bowel syndrome, inflammatory bowel disease, and bile malabsorption. If bile isn't produced properly or recycled by the liver, the entire gastrointestinal and digestive system can be thrown into a state of disease and malfunction.

Fat-Soluble Vitamin Storage/Metabolism

The human body requires a balance of different vitamins to maintain health and wellness. Common vitamins that people know about, usually due to a deficiency, are vitamins A, B, C, D, E, and K. There are many other vitamins that the human body needs, though.

Most vitamins can be consumed through foods and with a healthy, balanced diet. Others are taken in from the environment, like vitamin D, which can be absorbed through the eyes and skin from exposure to sunlight. If you've ever experienced a vitamin deficiency, you may have been told by a doctor or health care provider to take a dietary supplement that has concentrated portions of the vitamin you need more of. Whether it is through diet, supplements, or environmental factors, vitamins are taken into the body and are responsible for a lot of different chemical and physical processes in the body.

Vitamins A, D, E, and K are known as fat-soluble vitamins. This means that they are all soluble in organic solvents. They are also metabolized, transported, and absorbed in a similar way as fats. These fat-soluble vitamins are the ones that the liver ends up being responsible for.

Most fat-soluble vitamins travel to the liver from the intestines, where they are absorbed. Once in the liver, depending on the vitamin, its purpose in the body, and its molecular makeup, the liver will either metabolize the vitamin or store it.

Vitamin K is slightly different from its fat-soluble friends. Rather than being stored or metabolized in the liver, vitamin K is the liver enzyme that makes it vital to liver function.

Vitamin A deficiencies can lead to rashes, ocular disorders such as night blindness, and an impaired immune system. Vitamin D deficiencies can result in an increased risk of cardiovascular disease, rickets, asthma in children, cognitive impairment, and depression. Vitamin E deficiencies can lead to muscle weakness, walking and coordination problems, immune system problems, and trouble with vision, along with numbness and tingling. Vitamin K deficiencies have been known to result in excessive bleeding from cuts and wounds, easy bruising, heavy menstrual periods, oozing from the nose and gums, and blood in the urine or stool.

This list of deficiency-related health problems is to outline just how important vitamins are to the body and overall health. If your liver is overtaxed or in some way damaged, storing and metabolizing vitamins can become more difficult. Vitamin deficiencies aren't just caused by not consuming vitamin-rich foods, supplements, or being out in the environment. They can also be the result of the body not being able to process vitamins, which would stem from liver problems.

Drug Metabolism

A common treatment for a lot of different symptoms and ailments in modern-day medicine is the use of chemical drugs and pharmaceuticals. These drugs have an important role when it comes to bodily health. The liver also has an important function in how these medications and drugs interact with the body.

For these medications and drugs to be effective in the body, they have to undergo a metabolic process. This process helps to release their compounds into the body and allows the body to process the compounds and then gain the benefits from the medication. Since drugs are usually manufactured with some chemical components, they can have small doses of toxic particles that need to be filtered out of the body. If these particles aren't filtered out, they can build up and start to cause other problems.

The liver plays a major role in not only metabolizing drugs and medications but also in filtering out the waste and potentially toxic particles. Through a two-phase process, the liver can break down and metabolize the medications. The kidneys and gut are also helpful in drug metabolism.

When it comes to properly breaking down medications and filtering out the waste, many factors contribute to proper metabolic processes. Age, gender, interactions between drugs, pregnancy, diabetes, kidney disease, liver disease, genetics, and inflammation can also affect drug metabolism. In regards to liver health, a few of those factors can be lessened or soothed by having a healthy, strong liver.

Bilirubin Metabolism

Heme is a porphyrin class compound that contains iron. It forms the non-protein portion of hemoglobin and other biological molecules. Hemoglobin is a protein molecule in red blood cells. As a part of the red blood cells, hemoglobin is a very important protein molecule in the body. Heme is just as important, being a part of the hemoglobin makeup.

The liver is one organ that plays a major role in the breakdown of heme. Other organs that play a role in hemolysis, the breakdown of heme, include the spleen and bone marrow. The hemolysis process breaks heme down into biliverdin, which is further broken down into bilirubin. Once in the bilirubin form, it is secreted by bile through feces. Some bilirubin is reabsorbed by gut bacteria or to be a part of enterohepatic circulation.

This filtration process is important to the health of the blood and circulatory system. All cells in the body go through a process of use, function, and death, including blood cells. When a cell reaches the end of its life, it needs to be properly recycled or eliminated. The liver becomes that recycle-and-elimination catalyst for many kinds of cells in the body. This is how it plays a role in blood purification.

Other Functions

Other important functions of the liver include the thyroid hormone function and managing the synthesis of plasma proteins and clotting factors of all intrinsic and extrinsic pathways, except factor VIII.

The thyroid is an endocrine gland that is responsible for the production of a lot of hormones that are important to the body. These hormones impact the metabolism, internal body temperature, and growth and development of the body. Having the liver help regulate and manage thyroid hormone production is astronomically important to overall health and wellness.

Hopefully, you can now see how the liver plays its part in relation to other important systems and processes in the body. It has a role in bodily functions that are in completely different cavities of the body. An organ that has such strong relationships throughout the body should be respected and cared for.

A liver detox is considered one way to cleanse the liver and help to support the organ so that it can function at its optimal levels. However, there are lifestyle changes that are beneficial to long-term liver health. That means that once you have done your liver detox or cleanse, you'll want to take measures in your life with diet, exercise, and other healthy changes that will ensure your liver stays healthy long term.

As your liver strengthens over time, you'll see vast improvements in bodily health, and you might even see some chronic or long-term conditions beginning to clear up.

HOW TO KNOW IF A LIVER DETOX IS RIGHT FOR YOU

Before getting too deep into the concept of a liver detox, let's go over what the term "detox" means, what the goal of a detox is, and when and why you should go through a detox program. Before we can talk about detoxes, we need to first talk about toxins in the body.

What are toxins? "Toxin" is a somewhat blanket term that covers the buildup of any substance in the body that can result in health problems or unwanted side effects. Most of the time, the body can flush toxins out on its own. One of the components of these functions is the liver. Some of the common toxins that people are exposed to daily include caffeine, alcohol, heavy metals, pollutants, acids, bases, and medications.

When the body is functioning at optimal health, toxins don't have the chance to build up or cause problems. However, filtration and detox functions in the body can become impaired just from daily life. Exposure to certain types of foods, environmental factors, medications, and medical issues can result in an impairment of body filtration systems. When the toxins begin to build up, the body has to work twice as hard to filter them out.

If the buildup is a result of some sort of damage, such as a medical condition or long-term use of a medication, then your body might not be able to catch up with the toxin elimination. Additionally, if the body has to work twice as hard to remove toxins and keep up with continued exposure, the organs in your body begin to get overtaxed, like the liver. An overtaxed organ is less effective and can start to wear out or break down. This is why the liver can have lasting damage from the overconsumption of alcohol. It can't keep up with the filtration of toxins from alcohol consumption, which eventually pushes the liver into failure.

Just to be clear, a lot of the toxins that we are exposed to regularly are in harmless quantities. Heavy metals like lead, mercury, and cadmium as well as substances like arsenic are present in a lot of environmental ways, such as in the pesticides that are used commercially or in pollution from factories. Cigarette smoke is another source of these toxic substances, as is food, in some cases, especially certain kinds of fish that are high in mercury levels. In moderation and with the body filtering toxins out properly, these substances don't build up or cause problems.

Unfortunately, it is very easy in this day and age to have the body systems and organs struggle with their primary functions. This is in regards to the over-prescribing of medications, easy access to unhealthy junk food, the use of more potent and toxic pesticides, and an increase in environmental pollution. Overexposure to any of these substances can result in toxin buildup in the body. Some heavy metals, in excess, can even inhibit the systems and processes that are responsible for eliminating them. This serves to exacerbate the problem.

In some cases, heavy metals can compete with the natural absorption of minerals in the body. This leads to toxic buildups and an ever-increasing deficiency in the minerals that your body needs.

It is fair to say that toxin buildup in the body is not good and can result in a lot of health problems and concerns. So, the question becomes, how do you remove the toxins from your body?

Simple, a detox.

The liver is considered the second-hardest working organ in the body, after the ever-pumping heart. So, when you come to the conclusion that it is time for a detox cleanse, you should understand that the purpose of a detox is to help support the organs in your body that will filter out the toxins. With your liver, you want to offer enough support and relief that the liver can do its job without being overtaxed but also keep up with proper toxin filtration.

There are a lot of supplemental detox plans out on the market these days. They advertise a quick body flush and detox that will "reboot" your liver or other organs and systems. These detox programs advertise a fast way to lose weight, lower cholesterol, or repair the liver. While some of them may be effective, a true body detox and cleanse is a more involved commitment that extends beyond a single round of a supplemental detox.

A true detox program requires a commitment and willingness to change your lifestyle. You might not get immediate results, but the more you improve yourself and support your system, the more you will notice the changes in your body. This change can sometimes be subtle, but over time, it is hard to deny the benefits and the results.

You might not know it, but your liver could be giving you signs that you should pursue a detox program. A buildup of toxins in your system can result in mood changes, digestive problems, deteriorating organs, headaches, fatigue, infertility, reduced immune system function, problems with mental clarity, and tingling throughout the body. Other issues can present as unusual bloating, rapid and unexplained weight gain, trouble losing weight even with diet and exercise, changes in complexion or skin discoloration, heartburn, acid reflux, digestive issues, excessive perspiration, lack of internal homeostasis, and abnormal lipid panels. These are all potential signs that your liver is struggling to filter toxins from the body.

There are a few instances in which you might want to consider a detox program even if you haven't been experiencing any symptoms. If you are having trouble conceiving, are regularly exposed to poor quality air, work with metals or chemicals, have a house that was built before 1978, or live in a house with old, outdated plumbing, then you should consider a detox. These circumstances can result in toxin exposure, especially heavy metals. If you have concerns, you can even perform an at-home heavy metals blood test to see if there is a buildup of these toxic metals in your bloodstream.

It is worth noting that heavy metals are not the only kinds of toxins that can build up in your body. If you have any of the above symptoms or circumstances in your life, going through a liver detox program can help. Not only does it help to reduce toxin buildup in your body, but it can also help improve your overall health by introducing healthier habits into your lifestyle. This will prevent toxin buildups in the future and keep your organs functioning in a healthy way without overtaxing them.

2

NINE SIGNS YOUR LIVER IS UNHAPPY

Oftentimes, when the body is experiencing some kind of pain, discomfort, or ailment, it is just a symptom or sign of something else going on. These two terms—symptom and sign—are two terms that are going to be used regularly in this book when discussing livers and possible dysfunctions. In the medical field, a symptom is an unusual effect that is only felt or measurable from the perspective of the person feeling it. A sign is a measurable effect or visible effect in the body that can be observed by an outside source, like a medical professional.

For example, a headache would be considered a symptom because only the person experiencing the headache understands the pain, discomfort, or severity. A sign would be high blood pressure because this is a bodily state that can be measured and observed by medical equipment and blood tests.

While the medical field has advanced greatly over the past few hundred years, there have also been some setbacks. Medical professionals who have a specialty, such as osteopaths, radiologists, or neurosurgeons, get immersed in their field and sometimes lose sight of the big picture. This means that a patient can have a list of symptoms that they track, and a specialist might not be able to link them together if any of them impact body parts that don't coincide with their specialty.

Maybe you or someone you know has returned to a doctor again and again with a list of symptoms that deal with chronic pain, discomfort, digestion issues, or any number of other concerns. While these symptoms can be very telling about what is going on in the body, the modern medical field often discredits symptoms because they can't be measured. They look for signs of ailments or disease, and if they can't find any, they write off the patient, which can be frustrating.

With the way the medical field separates the body into so many different parts (e.g. skin, bones, joints, muscles, organs, hormones, and neurons), it can be hard to remember that all body parts are connected and that organs like the liver can be impacted by so many different bodily systems.

The medical field is always growing and evolving, and it is becoming clearer that there are flaws in the system with the deviation between signs and symptoms. A lot of people have encountered unsatisfactory experiences with medical professionals in recent years, and many have decided to turn to more holistic approaches. Holistic refers to an approach that treats the whole person or the whole body. This concept is what has paved the way for more information to come out in regards to liver detox plans and whole-body cleanses for health and wellness.

Let's look at an example of how a holistic approach can succeed. If a patient goes to their doctor with concerns about their thyroid, and the doctor determines that the thyroid isn't producing hormones correctly, the patient will likely be prescribed a medication to treat the thyroid or to make artificial thyroid hormones. However, as we discussed in Chapter

1, problems with the liver can impact the thyroid and hormone production. The medication might help balance the thyroid, but if the problem is in the liver, then it won't solve the issue, reverse it, or make it go away.

A holistic approach to thyroid problems would be to consider the body as a whole and look at what parts of the body can and do impact the thyroid separate from the gland itself. Then the whole body is treated with a focus on those parts that are directly related to the thyroid. So, when looking at a liver detox plan, it has a strong focus on the liver, but the methods implemented, like diet and exercise, are also targeted at the health and wellness of the entire body. This is what maintains the liver's functionality and keeps it healthy long-term.

The differences between modern medicine and holistic medicine are what result in the misinformation about the body. It is also why organs like the liver aren't discussed in general care or annual physicals. Just to clarify, there are plenty of situations where "what you see is what you get." That means that the symptoms and signs that have presented themselves are directly linked to the area they manifest in. However, this isn't always the case, especially in regards to chronic and recurrent conditions.

The other issue with signs and symptoms is that sometimes a lot of the same signs and symptoms can present themselves, but in two different people, they might be related to entirely different problems. This is another drawback to modern medicine. Doctors often have a definitive idea of how the body functions and what signs or symptoms correlate to specific ailments and diseases. This approach removes the creativity that is required for making unusual diagnoses as well as taking into consideration that all bodies are different and react and behave differently.

Since holistic medicine and treatments approach the body

as a whole, they are much more likely to analyze each symptom and sign as a separate entity to find the source. This helps to prevent misdiagnosis if the signs and symptoms aren't what are typically seen for the disease or problem.

Misdiagnosis is, unfortunately, not uncommon. Several years ago, a friend's daughter was experiencing severe knee pain. It was so bad she could hardly stand or walk. She had to go on medical leave from her job and was spending most of her days sitting or lying down. In her youth, she'd had a bilateral knee condition (both knees) in regards to her patella (kneecap). Her parents took her back to the osteopath who had treated the original knee condition.

The osteopath was a great doctor and a leader in his field. However, without even examining this young woman, he watched her walk across the room and proclaimed that it wasn't the same knee problem. So, he referred her to a rheumatologist thinking she had early-onset rheumatoid arthritis. Keep in mind that this journey started with this young woman going to her primary care physician, who referred her to the osteopath. It took over two weeks to get an appointment. Now, she had to wait another two and a half weeks to get in with the rheumatologist.

After over a month of being shuffled around and referred, she finally got her appointment. When the rheumatologist poked around at her kneecaps, he told her that she didn't have arthritis, that 23-year-olds don't get rheumatoid arthritis so suddenly, and that she was suffering from the same knee problem that had plagued her in her youth. The condition the osteopath so confidently dismissed.

This anecdote is a perfect example of how specialists can overlook signs that don't correspond to what they expect to see. The osteopath was so convinced that he was seeing a different condition based on the signs that had manifested, he didn't even do a physical exam on her knees. Fortunately, this young woman was able to get proper treatment for her knees, and she has lived comfortably for over five years without any relapses.

Since the liver has connections to so many organs, organ systems, and body functions, the same issue can come up with doctors if the liver is misbehaving or struggling. Modern medicine certainly has its place and its advantages, but one of the best ways you can help yourself is to take preventative measures for your entire body, especially for the organs that work so hard in your body, like the liver and heart.

SIGNS AND SYMPTOMS THAT MIGHT INDICATE YOUR LIVER IS STRUGGLING

As previously mentioned, there are no cut-and-dried signs or symptoms that absolutely indicate a problem with the liver. Short of a liver disease diagnosis, it can be difficult to pinpoint the cause of your signs and symptoms. That being said, there are some common indicators that the liver is struggling. This won't be the same for everyone, but on average, these are the nine major signs and symptoms that have been observed and reported.

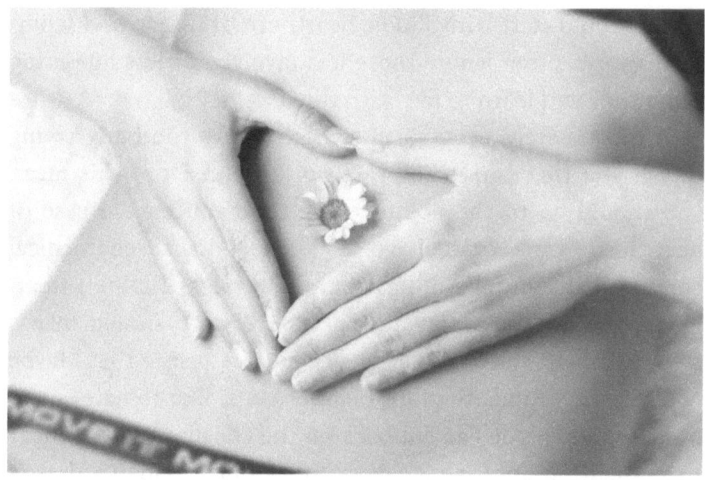

Let's take a look at what may indicate the liver is overtaxed and in need of a detox:

- Unexpected or rapid weight gain or an inability to lose weight with diet and exercise
- Unusual abdominal bloating (not related to other symptoms like the menstrual cycle)
- Heartburn
- Poor sleep
- Mysterious hunger or cravings
- Overheating of the body or a lack of internal homeostasis
- Changes in complexion or skin discoloration
- Sluggish liver
- Chemical sensitivities or allergies

Since an organ like the liver is so imperative to the body and bodily functions, when it starts to struggle, symptoms and signs won't be scarce. Toxins take a while to build up in the body, and over time, different signs and symptoms manifest. It could start with simple heartburn or digestive discomfort. People often ignore those less involved or less hindering symptoms and learn to live with them.

Unfortunately, even small symptoms are the body trying to tell you that something isn't quite right. Does this mean you should go to the doctor every time you have a case of heartburn? Unless you have an already diagnosed medical condition that results in heartburn and might be life-threatening, this isn't recommended. However, you should take a step back and think about what could be causing it. Maybe you're eating foods that are high in acids, like tomatoes and hot peppers. If you can cut back on the consumption of those high acid foods, your heartburn might show drastic improvement.

So, symptoms and signs are your body's way of communicating that something isn't quite right. If you are currently experiencing or have experienced any of the nine signs or symptoms mentioned in the above list, there is a chance that your liver needs to be cleansed and detoxed. An unhappy liver only gets unhappier. A common misconception is that if a sign or symptom is ignored and goes away, then the problem is resolved. This is untrue. Usually, all that means is that the body has found a way to compensate for the pain or discomfort.

Massage therapists see this all the time. A client might come to them for chronic foot pain. After several sessions, they might find the source of the pain is an old surgical scar on the back. Over the years, the client unconsciously adjusted how they walked and sat to compensate for the discomfort from the surgical scar. Eventually, the pain traveled from the back, down the legs, and into the feet where it settled and became chronic.

The same thing can happen with organs. If you are working on determining where your signs and symptoms originate from, a good starting point is to track them. You can use a notebook, cellphone app, or computer program to make a list of signs and symptoms. Then track when you notice them, how long they last, and the immediate stimulus that aggravated them (if you can determine the cause). Over time, you might see patterns that emerge, which can help you get closer to the root cause, such as an overtaxed liver.

Another option to consider is to partake in a liver cleanse program if any of the above signs or symptoms have made themselves known in your life. A liver detox diet plan isn't going to be harmful to your body if your liver doesn't need the extra support. It can only help. Now, making those adjustments in your life can result in a loss of free time and mean more work and effort. You might not be willing to take that leap without more concrete evidence that your liver is in need of some support.

That is also a valid position to take. If you aren't convinced, try tracking some of the signs and symptoms before jumping into a liver detox plan. At the end of this chapter, testing your liver will also be discussed as an additional method for determining if a liver detox plan is right for you. Please also keep in mind that the signs and symptoms above are just a handful of problems that can arise from an overtaxed liver.

THE CONNECTION BETWEEN LIVER DISEASE AND MENTAL HEALTH, DEPRESSION, AND ANXIETY

Going back to the difference between signs and symptoms, there is one medical field that is almost entirely based on symptoms felt and reported by patients. This medical field is also considered one of the most taboo fields. While awareness is growing around it, concepts like mental health, depression, and anxiety are still labeled with a great deal of stigma, ridicule, and skepticism.

Mental health is hard to track and trace because it varies so greatly from person to person and centers almost exclusively on invisible symptoms. There are still those in modern society who say "it is all in their head" or who are otherwise convinced mental health is an excuse or a made-up reason for people to behave a certain way to justify how they feel.

It is unfortunate that there is such controversy around mental health because there are a lot of conditions that have arisen out of the mental health field that have shown that the mind can impact the physical body, thought patterns, and behaviors. The mind works off of chemical secretions and electrical impulses. If those impulses and secretions are in any way impaired or imbalanced, then the mind can become unhealthy in the same way the body can become unhealthy if the liver isn't working properly.

Liver disease and its connection to mental health, depression, and anxiety has been noted across several medical and psychological communities. It has been observed that those who have liver disease are more prone to anxiety, depression, and other mental health conditions.

In fact, across younger populations, it has been observed that youth with liver disease or chronic liver problems show a much higher rate of depression and anxiety or stress. A study performed in 2016 at a liver transplant clinic in London showed that the common stressors included problems sleeping, lethargy, concerns about money, problems at school or work, anxiety, and low self-esteem (Samyn, 2020, para 8).

It is recommended that younger age groups who are undergoing treatment for liver disease or who have been through a liver transplant be given an additional holistic therapy that doesn't just treat the body but also helps to treat and heal the mind to prevent a rise in mental health conditions caused by chronic liver disease.

While this study was based on young adults who were already diagnosed with liver disease, there is also evidence to suggest that psychosocial stress plays a role in causing liver disease, more specifically chronic viral hepatitis. Hepatitis is a liver-attacking condition. It has long been observed that anyone being treated for chronic illness that results in a stressful life or emotional state or who experiences exposure to lots of stressors shows a dramatic decline in physical health. This idea that stress can be harmful to the immune system or even break down the body isn't entirely novel.

However, studies done more recently on animals and humans have shown clear, definitive links between stress and how it can contribute to the development of viral hepatitis. These same studies went on to show that stress can also aggravate the inflammatory nature of liver cirrhosis. Since the liver plays a role in the immune system and several of the inter- and intra-cellular mechanisms, stress to the body and emotions can cause a more rapid progression of liver pathologies (Vere et al., 2009).

You can see just how the liver can be impacted by stress and anxiety that is often perceived as "normal" in today's society. You can also see how, on the flip side, problems in the liver can contribute to the manifestation of mental health concerns, like depression. So, the way you treat your body and live your life can have a direct impact on your liver, resulting in liver disease. Also, mild mental health conditions can be a sign or symptom that your liver is starting to struggle and no longer able to keep up with your lifestyle.

Speaking from a holistic approach, everything in the body is connected. Whether it is through connective tissue, the nervous system, or blood flow, the body is all connected. Even anxiety, depression, and responses to stress are your body's way of saying something isn't quite right. In a society where we are almost encouraged to stress ourselves out on a daily basis working grueling jobs, keeping up with family and community, balancing chores with friends, trying to squeeze in some personal time, and paying bills on time, stress becomes a major health factor for the body.

Some of what you are going to discover when learning about the liver detox and diet program is how to manage stress to help prevent it from becoming a problem for your liver. Additionally, if you have struggled with depression and anxiety throughout your life, you might want to add that to your symptom or sign list of reasons you should pursue a liver detox program.

TEST YOUR LIVER

If you need definitive proof before deciding to embark on a lifestyle change that will become your long-term liver detox and health plan, then you can consider having your liver tested for issues.

There are some at-home blood tests you can take to check on the status of your liver. Some, like Thorne's Heavy Metal At-Home Blood Test, might show a presence of heavy metals in the blood.

Various tests measure a variety of things, including levels of:

- Alanine transaminase (ALT)
- Aspartate aminotransferase (AST)
- Alkaline phosphatase (ALP)
- Albumin
- Bilirubin

When you go to the doctor, you might need a more

comprehensive exam specific to the liver to determine if anything is wrong. This could include a biological exam, ultrasound of the liver, or a hepatic biopsy. While these tests and examination procedures tend to be in regards to serious signs and symptoms, you can find at-home blood test kits that will screen for the listed items above.

If you do have serious concerns about your liver, try an at-home blood test. You might want to consult a qualified medical professional depending on the results. Or, you might decide that it is time for you to make the commitment to a liver detox diet plan.

3
INTRODUCTION TO THE LIVER DETOX PROGRAM

If you've been looking around for information about a liver detox, you've probably encountered a lot of different information about the pros and cons of detoxing, some medical information that might seem contradictory, and several different paths you can take to achieve your detox goals.

Like in most situations, there are a lot of different ways to go about meeting your goals. A lot of the liver detox and cleanse programs around, especially the ones that include supplements and strict fasting or "deep cleansing" methods, are meant for a short-term liver flush and reboot. The liver detox plan that was designed and built for this book is for long-term liver health. It does start with a short-term deep cleanse, but the overall intention is to provide a lifestyle changing plan that will support your liver for many years to come.

Just to clarify, the supplement detoxes and their quick-flush methods might be effective for some people and could be the overall goal. In the short term, they can be quite useful. However, "flushing" the body of toxins over three days or one week doesn't change the number of toxins that are entering your body on a daily basis due to your lifestyle and what you are exposed to environmentally.

Short-term liver flushes can become problematic for the body if used consistently as a way to diminish toxin buildup. Between the fasting and very specific dietary requirements, they aren't designed to manage toxin buildup in the body. A short-term detox or cleanse is designed to rid your body of accumulated toxins so you can start with a clean slate. Once the slate is clean, though, if you go back to the same habits as before, it will become gunked up with toxins again.

This is what sets this liver detox program apart.

This liver detox and cleansing program is meant to flush toxins from your system and also control the number of toxins that are put into your body regularly. Since there are so many different sources of toxins, like air pollution, bad drinking water, and lead paint in an old house, you won't be able to control every single toxic element that you are exposed to, but you don't have to.

A long-term liver support program begins with a quick flush but then also provides information, details, and step-by-step instructions on lifestyle changes that allow you to limit your toxin intake and thus protect your body from toxin buildups. This liver detox program takes it one step further by bringing in the holistic approach of supporting the body, mind, and emotions while you are detoxing and striving for a healthier future.

WHAT IS A LIVER DETOX?

A liver detox is simply a way to flush toxins out of your body, specifically the liver. It's typically not a complicated process, although it does require effort on your part. Hopefully, after reading the first two chapters, you understand the signs and symptoms that could allude to needing a liver cleanse. If you're still reading, you've probably decided a liver cleanse is right for you, but you may be wondering why this program and what the specific benefits are. Some of the benefits of liver detoxes have been touched on before, but below is a comprehensive list of the benefits to a liver detox program and long-term liver support.

A liver detox:

- Naturally boosts energy (no more relying on caffeine!)
- Removes bags and dark circles from under the eyes and reduces the redness and puffiness around the eyes
- Clears skin (this goes for acne, blotches, eczema, contact dermatitis, and other skin conditions that are perceived as topical)
- Normalizes the metabolism (which includes food processing, nutrient extraction, and bowel movements)
- Normalizes body weight to a healthy degree
- Brings blood cholesterol levels to a healthy zone
- Removes tongue coating, improving the sense of taste
- Helps support the immune system so it can better keep your body healthy and safe from pathogens, infections, viruses, and bacteria
- Reduces swellings and edemas (fluid buildups) in the body
- Keeps the body from bruising easily

These benefits, in turn, have other impacts on the body. For example, regulating metabolism, digestion, and body weight can be an important part of managing type 2 diabetes.

While type 2 diabetes may always require insulin use, managing body weight, metabolism, and digestion can reduce the amount of insulin that is required daily, also saving money in the long run.

If you have chronic skin conditions that don't seem to have a "root" cause, then it could be due to toxin buildups in the body. Acne is an increasingly common topical skin problem where the source is often unknown. Teenagers and adults can struggle with acne. No matter how much you wash your face, take acne medication, or reduce your sugar intake, you may still struggle, and the liver could be the culprit. If the liver isn't properly clearing the body of toxins, they manifest in other ways, such as acne, eczema, and other skin conditions. Despite the epidermis being on the outside of the body, if the interior of the body isn't functioning properly, then the exterior will show symptoms.

Many people struggle with weight loss. They go through cycles of diets and exercise and end up not making any progress. Sometimes, it isn't about targeting weight loss specifically. Just like with the skin conditions, the inability to lose weight can be a byproduct of an unhappy liver.

When it comes to a healthy immune system, the world is full of pathogens. They come as viruses, bacteria, infections, and diseases. The body's own defense system against these foreign invaders that seek to harm it is the immune system. With a healthy immune system, your body will be much better at fighting off these pathogens. Even if you get exposed, you will stand a better chance of not developing symptoms or having severe reactions because your body is able to keep the pathogens from causing damage.

That being said, there are known pathogens that are incredibly strong or new, and the body doesn't recognize them as dangerous and can't fight them off. A healthy immune system doesn't mean you aren't at risk of getting sick; it just means you might not get sick as often or the symptoms won't be as severe.

There are many benefits to a liver detox plan. The provided list is simply an introduction to what a liver detox can do for you.

A WORD OF WARNING

A word of caution before you jump into the first liver cleanse you see.

It is not uncommon these days to go into the health section of a grocery store, supplement store, or all-natural market and see advertisements for full detox programs. You can buy a detox box costing $50 or more that includes several supplements and instructions on how to complete the detox program. These boxes are generally only equipped with enough supplements to last for a few days to a week, giving the impression that once the supplements are gone, the detox is complete.

Unfortunately, a true cleanse that will greatly benefit the body is a long-term commitment. Fixing years' worth of stress and damage to the liver can't be resolved in just a few days. So, be wary of detox plans and programs that advertise "complete health" or "complete detox" in just a few days. Sometimes, these cleansing programs will go as far as to say that you'll see a drastic difference in your weight, clarity of skin, and other common concerns. Those are very attractive marketing methods, but without proper follow-up, they aren't going to manifest.

The other downside to a liver detox in a box is that some companies use quantities of supplements that can be harmful to the body or other organs or systems in the body. Some programs call for drinking large amounts of juices. This can be dangerous to anyone with diabetes or kidney disease.

Fasting is often a part of the detox-in-a-box plan. If done incorrectly, fasting can lead to weakness and fainting. Additionally, if you have liver damage from hepatitis B, fasting can make the damage worse. Even though the supplemental detox in a box idea is all-natural and doesn't include pharmaceuticals or heavy drugs, they are operating from the mentality of instant gratification and instant fixes.

A liver detox is more than a three- to seven-day cleansing program. It is more than just detox supplements and drinks. It is not a one-time program that fixes everything. This can be hard to accept sometimes because, in the age of technology and western medicine, instant gratification is the desired outcome when someone tries something new or wants to see a change. True change comes from practice and commitment, though. A true liver detox program is a lifestyle change with the desire to be healthy and support your liver function.

WHAT IS OUR LIVER DETOX PROGRAM?

Our liver detox program is going to start you off with a seven-day liver flush. The flush is primarily going to be based on diet and fasting; however, it is also going to cover some meditation techniques to help you maintain your mental and emotional health while your body is detoxing. You will also be given some simple exercise plans that are designed to boost your metabolism and natural energy. They won't be too intense or rigorous as your body is likely going to feel weak from the periods of fasting.

These seven days are going to be your first step toward liver health. The main goal of this flush is essentially to give your liver a break. It is designed to clear your body of toxins quickly and then greatly limit the number of toxins entering your body at that time so your liver can rest and reboot.

When your computer is a bit sluggish, tech support always recommends rebooting the computer as a first step. It is how your computer unloads all the "junk" files or unnecessary buildup of data that is dragging down the internal processing. In terms of your liver, the first seven-day flush is meant to do just that!

After the seven-day liver flush, you will have three days of meal plans, exercise, and meditation practices that will focus on building your liver's health and helping to repair any damage done to your liver before bringing it back to full function. These three days will primarily be focused on three meals a day, with a few snacks, that are solely designed for liver health.

So, after your liver is rebooted and your body is free of toxins, you want your liver to ease back into what has to be done. Consider this like rehab or recovery for your liver. If you've ever broken a bone in an arm or leg or had major surgery, then you know that during the recovering process, there is an element of physical therapy or rehab. Your body essentially needs to be reminded how to use that limb or body part once the long recovery period is over. If your liver has been struggling for a while, you'll need to remind it what it feels like to function normally. In doing so, you strengthen and prepare it to come back to full use, the same as you would a recovered broken leg. Fortunately, since the liver is an organ that doesn't require conscious effort to make it function, three days of rehab should be plenty to get it back into the swing of normality.

Once your three days of rejuvenation have ended, you will be given long-term instructions for maintaining liver health. These long-term plans will cover your diet with suggested regular meals and snacks. It will also cover proper exercise plans and strategies for keeping yourself healthy and maintaining your weight goals. You'll also be given additional meditation practices that are going to continue to foster a healthy and positive mindset toward your lifestyle changes and your personal health.

The long-term aspect of maintaining liver health is meant to be a lifelong practice. Keeping your liver healthy indefinitely is going to act as a great preventative in later life. With age, the body naturally becomes more susceptible to health conditions. If your liver is kept strong and healthy, your body will be less susceptible to age-related breakdowns of the immune system and other organ functions. It is not a solution for aging, just a solution for long-term health and wellness.

There will be a section of the detox plan that covers meals for your whole family if you're looking to keep everyone in your household healthy as well. The step-by-step instructions provided will also include helpful information about why these steps and methods are implemented in regards to liver flushing, detoxing, and long-term liver health.

During the seven-day flush, there will be recommendations for liver-supporting supplements that can be taken. The supplements that are recommended are going to be safe, and they will include any precautions to consider before taking them. They aren't necessary to our liver detox program; however, they can help facilitate the process and help your liver rebound a bit faster.

It is important to make the distinction between these recommended dietary supplements and the liver detox in a box. Individual supplements, like milk thistle, are a pure source of that herb. The same is true of supplements like omega-3s and minerals like zinc. They aren't a blend or combination. They are capsuled out with healthy proportions and have instructions for proper daily usage. They are also entirely optional for your use.

Before you get started with your liver detox program, it is recommended that you get a notebook or journal to dedicate to your plan. If it is easier to keep an electronic record of what you do and experience, find a good phone app or computer program that will allow you to track your progress.

Not only can you use this journal to keep notes on what you are supposed to be doing at which stage of the detox plan you are in, but you can also use it to track changes in your body. Recording specific feelings, sensations, and anything you notice is a good way to track the subtle changes that might go unnoticed. It can be very motivating to have notes in black and white that validate and confirm your progress.

This notebook serves a dual purpose, though. If some parts of the program don't work for you or some work very well, you'll notice and be able to adjust your plan accordingly. You'll be able to gradually phase out things that don't benefit you and replace them with things that do. Everyone's body is different, and you might not have the same success with certain methods. That's perfectly okay. Additionally, if you have any specific allergies or preexisting conditions, you might need to shift and alter the plan so that it remains healthy for you.

You can keep track of more than just what happens to your body physically. You can also write down the thoughts and feelings you have during the detox program. When your body begins to detox, you'll likely experience mood swings or changes in mood. Writing about them can help you to manage them as well as reflect on what you felt as you moved through the program. Since there is a meditation aspect to this detox program, writing about thoughts, feelings, and experiences from the meditations will enhance the holistic side of the program.

Notebooks and journals, especially if they are electronic, are easily portable. That means you can keep them with you even if you can't keep this book with you. If you keep track of your step-by-step plan in your notebook, there aren't any excuses for not following the plan.

CHECK WITH YOUR DOCTOR BEFORE STARTING A CLEANSE

Prior to committing to or starting our liver detox program, you should check in with your primary doctor or health care professional. If you have any preexisting conditions, this is vitally important. There are some conditions that can't handle a liver detox, especially when there is a fasting or juice/smoothie component, as our program includes.

People with kidney disease and diabetes should definitely handle the juice intake of a liver detox program carefully and only with the consent and moderation of a doctor. If you have any kidney disease or known damage, proceed with caution and only with the express permission of a qualified healthcare provider. Some kidney diseases and damage can be aggravated by the detox program steps.

It is important to know what a liver detox and long-term health plan can do for you, but since long-term health is the overall goal, you want to do it right. If you're prone to food allergies, be careful with the recipes if they include foods you haven't eaten before. You might need to make substitutions to the recipes, but be sure to use complementary ingredients that won't disrupt the cleanse or detox program.

Anyone with low blood pressure, low iron, or a history of fainting should be careful of the fasting portions and consult a doctor or health care professional to make sure fasting is safe for them. Additionally, if you're pregnant, for your health and your baby's health, you might consider holding off on the detox program until after your baby is born, unless your doctor gives you the go-ahead.

A preexisting condition doesn't automatically exclude you

from being able to perform or benefit from our liver detox program. You want to make sure that it is going to benefit you though, and that is why anyone, even someone without a preexisting condition, should double-check with their physician before starting. Your health is the overall goal, so make sure you stand to gain benefits before starting.

Once you've done that, it's time to get started.

4

A LIVER DETOX PROGRAM THAT WILL LEAVE YOU FEELING ENERGIZED AND HEALTHY

Welcome to the first steps of your liver detox program. To begin, you'll start with a somewhat intensive liver flush that will span seven days. For a whole week, you'll want to stick to this step-by-step program to ensure that your body is flushed of toxins and your liver is ready to refresh and work toward making you healthier.

You'll notice that the seven-day flush is broken down by day. Each day is going to cover an outline of what you should be doing for your flush on those days. This program isn't meant to disrupt your daily life. You might need to make some timing adjustments to work in the meditations and the exercise portions. However, overall, you won't need to put your life on hold or change your daily schedule.

Like the seven-day flush, the three-day rejuvenation plan has also been broken down into specific days with clear instructions on how to handle your liver on those days. The three days are a little more demanding when it comes to exact meals because it is based on a plan that was developed by a cirrhosis patient. You might want to double-check your kitchen to make sure you have the necessary equipment or substitute equipment for the food preparation that comes with this liver support plan.

Even if you don't have a lot of experience cooking, it is recommended that you begin your own meal prep or ask for the assistance of someone in your house or a friend or family member who can cook to help teach you. Part of the liver detox plan is to monitor what is going into your body. Purchasing premade foods or ordering takeout from restaurants isn't going to have the same food quality, even if the menu item looks or sounds identical to what you should be preparing.

Please remember that while you are detoxing, your body might go through a lot of changes. Your moods might be a little more complicated or tumultuous. Overall, by the end of the intensive detox, you should feel more energized, healthier, and more positive.

SEVEN-DAY LIVER FLUSH

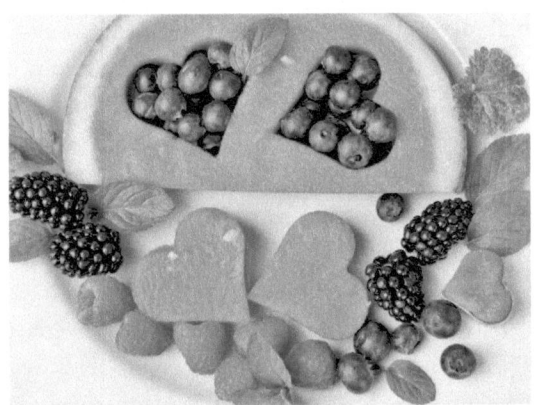

To ensure that your liver flush is effective, there are some dos and don'ts to cover so that you are fully prepared for the process. First and foremost, you'll want to review the information about what to eat and drink. Then, stock up your kitchen with the goodies that you can eat and drink for your cleanse. If it is an option, you might even want to remove those items you can't eat and drink for the duration of your week-long flush. This will help to avoid the temptation to break from your flush diet.

Important "don'ts" for your seven-day flush include:

- Don't eat wheat and gluten. They are both gut irritants. Give your digestive system a week-long break.
- Don't eat milk and dairy. Milk is a common food allergen, and the body creates antibodies for it, stimulating and overtaxing your immune system. Milk also prompts the body to create more mucus. After a week without dairy, you might even find that you feel so good you don't want to reintroduce it.
- Don't consume caffeine. As hard as it is not to have your morning coffee or that afternoon cup of black tea, try to avoid it because caffeine is contributing to your liver's overtaxation. Caffeine is an addictive toxin that the liver works hard to flush out. Use this as an opportunity to kick the habit and restore your liver. **Tip:** If you absolutely cannot cut caffeine out of your daily life, stick to no more than two cups of green tea a day. Green tea is full of antioxidants, which are important during a cleanse, and isn't super high in caffeine content. It is a fine line, so only walk it if there are no other options.
- Don't drink alcohol. This is huge when it comes to liver detoxing and liver health. Alcohol is arguably

your liver's greatest enemy. Cut it out for a week to truly let your liver rest.
- Don't consume processed sugars and processed foods. When possible, avoid foods with sugars and sweeteners that aren't natural. Raw honey and pure maple syrup are unprocessed, natural sugars. You can substitute them for other sugars if you'd like. Consuming lots of sugary foods and processed foods heavy in preservatives can counteract what you are trying to do as sugar bogs down your energy levels and processed foods are a lot harder to digest, contributing to excess weight.
- Don't smoke cigarettes or vape. The chemicals in cigarette smoke and vaping juice interfere with the detox program. Plus, they are bad for you and will cause other long-term problems.
- Don't eat a lot of saturated fat. Saturated fat and barbecued meat are also inhibitors to the liver flush process. Be conscientious of the amount of saturated fat you are consuming, and stay away from the charcoal grill during your detox.

A few "dos" or habits to pick up while you are working on your seven-day liver flush include:

- Drink water consistently throughout the day. It will help keep wastes and fluids moving through your system and get them eliminated from your body. Staying hydrated will also help to facilitate the process. **Tip**: Drinking more water inevitably leads to more bathroom breaks. Plan accordingly whenever possible.
- Eat superfoods. These will be covered in more detail shortly.

Fruits that you'll want to eat plenty of during your detox include fresh apricots, cantaloupe, kiwi, peaches, papaya, citrus fruits, melons, red grapes, mangoes, and berries of all kinds. Vegetables that will benefit your detox plan include peppers, beets, broccoli, artichokes, red cabbage, Brussels sprouts, cauliflower, carrots, kale, pumpkin, cucumber, spinach, sweet potatoes, watercress, tomato, and bean and seed sprouts.

These are the superfoods. All of the above foods are high in antioxidants, vitamins, protein, minerals, healthy starches, healthy fats, and substances like chlorophyll that helps to leech heavy metals and toxins from the body.

There are other foods that you can eat during a detox program, but they should be consumed in moderation. Limit your grain intake, and stick to whole grains that are gluten-free (e.g. brown rice, quinoa, and oats). Limit your fish consumption to no more than once daily. Stick to fish like salmon, mackerel, anchovies, and sardines that are known to be lower in mercury than other popular fish such as tuna and swordfish.

During the seven days of detoxing, you can have one serving every other day of foods like bananas and potatoes. They have starches and chemicals that imitate hormones like estrogen. These types of foods need to be consumed with care during a detox.

Nuts and seeds should be consumed daily but in a single quantity of roughly one handful. They are rich in natural, good fats and proteins. Nuts and seeds to eat include Brazil nuts, almonds, pecans, hazelnuts, sunflower seeds, pumpkin seeds, flaxseed, chia seeds, and sesame seeds. You'll want to consider switching to extra virgin olive oil as a cooking oil and using flaxseed oil or another cold-pressed seed oil for cold oil bases (like salad dressings).

There are foods to completely avoid during your liver

detox flush as well. As mentioned above, avoid all milk and dairy, including cheese, yogurt, ice cream, and cream. You should also avoid meat during these seven days. Red meat, chicken and poultry, pork, eggs—take a break from all meat for seven days. Grains like rye, wheat, spelt, and barley all have gluten in them, so avoid those grains as well.

Additionally, you shouldn't be consuming salt during this seven-day flush. Avoid foods that have sodium. Stay away from hydrogenated fats, preservatives, artificial sweeteners, and processed sugars, as well as fried foods, spices, and dried fruits.

It seems like a lot to keep track of, but the seven-day breakdown below gives you the steps to utilize this information in a healthy way.

Optional: Supplements that you can take during your seven-day cleanse include a multivitamin and a comprehensive antioxidant supplement. The superfoods and the diet suggestions for your seven-day plan all include high levels of vitamins, minerals, and antioxidants. It isn't necessary to take them, but they can give your flush and liver an added boost.

Antioxidants combat the body's internal and external exposure to oxidants. Oxidants, in abundance, can cause cell damage, triggering many conditions such as inflammation and even cancer. Regardless of whether or not you're doing a liver cleanse, antioxidants are important to health and wellness. However, a proper, balanced diet gets you those vitamins and antioxidants without the aid of supplements.

Some other optional liver-supporting supplements include milk thistle extract, dandelion extract, glutamine, and MSM. Milk thistle extract binds to toxins to help remove them from the body and increases glutathione to keep toxins moving through the body until they are eliminated.

MSM is a sulfur compound. It is a liver-supporting compound that also aids in the production of glutathione.

Dandelion extract has been used for centuries in various herbal remedies and by herbalists. While it is commonly considered a weed, it is also a very beneficial plant. Dandelion extract supports the liver and also helps with the production of bile. Bile, as outlined in Chapter 1, plays a major role in liver function and detoxifying the body.

If you decide to take any vitamins and supplements, double- and triple-check the dosage and usage instructions on the bottle. Also, look for any potential contraindications and conflicts with preexisting conditions. If you don't see any obvious notes but have a preexisting condition, consult your doctor or primary care physician to determine the safety of taking these supplements. Be mindful of the fact that our liver program doesn't require the use of any vitamins or supplements to work.

When a cleanse refers to "fasting," it doesn't mean to avoid food for long periods. This kind of fasting is in relation to cutting out processed and unhealthy foods and sticking to raw, healthy foods such as light fruits and vegetables, as described above. Quantities of food are shrunk down as well.

In the breakdown of each day, there will be specific recipes referenced. The actual recipes, along with others that aren't referenced specifically, that can be included in your liver flush and rejuvenation plans will be included in the bonus chapter of this book. The benefits of each superfood will be included in parentheses, so feel free to choose the one that fits your needs best.

Meditations will also be mentioned, and the instructions for these meditations will also be included in the "recipes" bonus chapter. Use the notes in that chapter to follow along and perform the meditation properly.

A helpful tip for starting your seven-day flush is to begin on a weekend day, like a Saturday, so you can practice getting in the swing without job expectations. This gives you some time to adjust to this new plan.

DAY 1

Start your day off with one of the following cleansing, detoxifying beverages:

- Cucumber-mint detox
- Orange, carrot, and ginger detox

Follow up your detox beverage with a small bowl of mixed fresh berries. Any combination will do:

- Blueberries
- Strawberries
- Raspberries
- Gooseberries
- Goji berries
- Blackberries
- Acai berries
- Cranberries
- Grapes

For lunch, enjoy a warm cup of dandelion tea with raw honey (liver and bile support, a natural sweetener that helps with seasonal allergies).

Have yourself a handful of nuts and seeds (high in protein, healthy fats, healthy oils, and antioxidants). Mix any of the following nuts and seeds:

- Pecans

- Hazelnuts
- Brazil nuts
- Almonds
- Pumpkin seeds
- Sunflower seeds
- Chia seeds
- Flaxseeds
- Sesame seeds

Also, eat a fresh apricot and carrot sticks with your nuts and seeds (antioxidants, detoxing, and healthy) and a detoxifying "drink your greens" fruit and vegetable juice (full of vitamin K and other essential vitamins).

Take a five-minute walk outside (weather permitting). If you can't walk outside and there is no convenient indoor area to take a five-minute walk (indoor track, gym, shopping mall), try doing five minutes of gentle stretches at home.

For dinner, eat something filling but light:

- Herb and mushroom rice casserole
- Artichoke heart and bean salad
- Potato, leek, and bean soup

After dinner, set 10 to 15 minutes aside for the Gratitude Meditation. The first few days of detoxing can be rough on the body and make you feel worse in some cases. It is important to give thanks to and remember what you have to be grateful for so that you focus more on gratitude and less on what your body is feeling. This can help prevent you from abandoning the cleanse.

DAY 2

Begin your day with a detoxifying beverage:

- Lemona (boosts energy naturally)
- Pomegranate and beet juice (boosts immune system)

After your beverage, fix yourself a bowl of mixed melon. Include any of the following:

- Watermelon
- Honeydew
- Cantaloupe
- Muskmelon

Also, enjoy a small portion of cinnamon porridge with your mixed melon.

At lunchtime, treat yourself to an antioxidant smoothie:

- Almond banana bread (good source of antioxidants; potassium; vitamins A, C, and K; and a good source of omega-3 fatty acids)
- Honey mint (full of minerals like copper and magnesium, also good against seasonal allergies)

To complete your lunch, add in an artichoke heart and bean salad.

In the afternoon, take another five-minute walk outside, weather permitting. If the weather is poor or you do not have a decent indoor location for walking, do some basic stretches or throw some music on and dance like no one is watching for 5 to 10 minutes. Dancing freely can be quite liberating in many ways!

With your dinner, drink a cup of dandelion tea with raw honey. Have yourself some Dijon salmon with steamed veggies and wild rice.

When your day is winding down, set aside 10 to 15 minutes for another Gratitude Meditation. Keeping yourself in good spirits and focused on what you are grateful for will continue to give you the mental and emotional stability to push through the discomfort of the first few days of fasting and detoxing.

DAY 3

Before eating breakfast, treat yourself to a cleansing, detoxifying beverage:

- Cucumber-mint detox
- Orange, carrot, and ginger detox

For breakfast, have a bowl of berry and seed porridge.

At lunchtime, drink a cup of dandelion tea with the fresh-squeezed juice from a slice of lemon and some raw honey. Eat a cup of carrot and lentil soup with a fresh apricot on the side and a handful of mixed nuts and seeds.

Sometime between lunch and dinner, make time to take a 10- to 15-minute walk outside. This walk should not be intense or rigorous. It is meant to be a casual stroll so you don't overextend your body or energy. While fasting and cleansing, you might feel dizzy or weak, but daily exercise is still important. Take it slow and don't overextend yourself until you feel pain or cause injury. If the weather is lousy, find an indoor location to walk for 10 to 15 minutes.

Dinner on the third day can be olive basmati rice with a detoxifying "drink your greens" fruit and vegetable juice.

Close your day out with a 15-minute Mindfulness Meditation to help you reconnect with your body. At this point, you'll be starting to come out of the lousy, crummy, almost sluggish feeling of the detox flush. Shifting your mentality to be more connected to your body is going to help you feel that changes are happening so you can understand the progress this program is providing.

DAY 4

Start your day with a detoxifying flush beverage:

- Lemona
- Pomegranate and beet juice

For breakfast, enjoy an antioxidant smoothie:

- Almond banana bread
- Smoothie verde (high in vitamin C and other essential vitamins)

With your smoothie, enjoy a cup of essential seed porridge.

For lunch, try one of these cleansing salads:

- Salmon fillet salad
- Rainbow trout salad
- Anchovy salad

Drink a cup of detoxifying juice rich in vitamins, minerals, and antioxidants.

During the afternoon, set aside 10 to 15 minutes for a walk outside. If the weather isn't good for an outdoor walk, find an indoor location. At this point in your cleanse, energy should be returning. At the very least, your body won't feel so weak anymore because it is adjusting to the new foods and smaller portions. If you want to take a more purposeful walk, start slow and don't overdo it. You can begin a power walking regime while taking precautions against dehydration and overworking yourself.

Eat a light and filling meal for dinner:

- Rice-stuffed peppers with salad
- Super quinoa salad

With your dinner, drink a cup of dandelion tea flavored with raw honey and a spritz of fresh lemon juice from a slice of lemon.

To relax at the end of your day, set 10 to 15 minutes aside for the Deep Breathing Meditation. Keeping your breath strong and your body vitalized with oxygen will have a major impact on your flush along with the increase in exercising.

DAY 5

To start day five of your liver flush, enjoy a detoxifying beverage:

- Cucumber-mint detox
- Orange, carrot, and ginger detox

Have an apple or a pear with a handful of nuts and seeds. Drink a glass of "drink your greens" cleansing juice with your breakfast.

At lunch, drink a cup of dandelion tea with raw honey and the fresh lemon juice from one lemon slice.

For your meal, have either:

- Potato, leek, and bean soup

- Herb and mushroom rice casserole.

On the side, eat a fruit salad made of mixed melons and antioxidant-rich berries.

In the afternoon, take a 15-minute walk outside, weather permitting. Or find an indoor location where you can walk for 15 minutes. If your energy levels are up for it, stick to power walking so you can boost your metabolism and work toward a healthy body weight.

For dinner, try one of these leafy, vitamin-rich, cleansing salads:

- Artichoke heart and bean salad
- Rainbow trout salad

When you've finished dinner and are getting ready to wrap up your day, set 10 to 15 minutes aside for a meditation practice. On your fifth day, you'll be returning to the Gratitude Meditation. Even though your body is getting used to the adjustments you've made for the flush, gratitude is a very important mindset to foster, especially in keeping up with and maintaining your liver health long term.

DAY 6

Begin your day with a flush beverage to detox:

- Lemona
- Pomegranate and beet juice

Enjoy one of the porridge options for breakfast:

- Cinnamon porridge
- Berry and seed porridge

- Essential seed porridge

Also, treat yourself to an antioxidant smoothie:

- Almond banana bread
- Honey mint
- Smoothie verde

For lunch, have a glass of sweet carrot fruit and vegetable juice (high in vitamins, minerals, and antioxidants). Eat a bowl of mixed melon along with a chickpea and sesame seed salad.

Before dinner and after lunch, make time to take a 15-minute walk, preferably outside but inside if the weather isn't ideal. Stick to walking, even if you want to quicken the pace a bit. With any kind of fasting cleanse, it is not recommended that you push yourself to jog or run, even if you feel like your energy levels are "back to normal." Part of a fasting cleanse is to reduce your caloric intake, which means your body won't be in a state for harder exercising.

With your dinner, drink a cup of dandelion tea with a spritz of fresh lemon juice and some raw honey. Whip yourself up some Thai-style snapper for a delicious detox meal.

Relax with a 10- to 15-minute Deep Breathing Meditation to wrap up your day and slow down your body, mind, and emotions.

DAY 7

On the last day of your intense flush, begin your day with a detoxifying beverage:

- Cucumber-mint detox
- Orange, carrot, and ginger detox

For breakfast, have a nice fruit salad with mixed berries, melons, and apples. Accompany your fruit salad with a handful of mixed nuts and seeds.

At lunchtime, drink a cup of dandelion tea flavored with a bit of fresh-squeezed lemon juice and raw honey. Eat a cup of soup for lunch:

- Carrot and lentil soup
- Potato, leek, and bean soup

Also, enjoy a fresh apricot, mango, or kiwi with your soup.

Give yourself 20 minutes between lunch and dinner to take a walk outside. If the weather isn't nice enough for an outdoor walk, find somewhere indoors where you can have a nice 20-minute walk. Movement and blood flow are both vital to health and detoxing. Both keep fluids and waste moving through your body until they can be eliminated. When you sweat, you release toxins through your pores, and this is a good way to naturally increase your energy levels. Still stick to casual walking or power walking. You won't want to embark on a more rigorous workout plan until after your seven-day flush.

With your dinner, drink a glass of sweet carrot juice. Eat one of the light-yet-filling meal options:

- Super quinoa salad
- Rice-stuffed peppers with salad
- Dijon salmon with wild rice and steamed veggies

When your day is winding down, do another 15 minutes of Mindfulness Meditation to reconnect with your body. You might be surprised to notice changes since the last time you did this meditation. Connecting with your body in this manner helps you form a healthier attachment and relationship to yourself and your physical body, and that goes a long way toward long-term health and maintaining health and wellness.

THREE-DAY LIVER REJUVENATION

You did it! You made it through the seven-day intense liver fasting flush! At this point in the program, your liver has been given a week-long break from all the things that can be consumed and cause problems for it. You might even be able to feel major changes in your body as far as natural energy levels, improvements in mood, feelings of clarity, and clearer skin. These are all fantastic accomplishments! Even if you can't see any noticeable changes, the simple fact that you made it through is a great accomplishment in its own right.

Now comes the three-day program where you will be rehabbing your liver. This vital organ has been given a nice break. Now, it is time to remind it how to function in a healthy way and keep up with what is being put in your body. When it comes to this rejuvenation period, you'll want to stick to the same recommendations of what to avoid as were laid out in the above section.

A lot of the foods, drinks, and standards are still the same during this three-day period. You don't want to bring back substances like alcohol, dairy, and meat before your liver has a chance to recharge and rejuvenate. You will, however, have more leniency when it comes to adding snacks, desserts, larger portions of food, and even different kinds of exercise into the rejuvenation process. Your body and liver have been flushed. Now it is time to get the liver back on track.

For all three days, begin with a detoxifying beverage:

- Lemona
- Cucumber-mint detox

- Pomegranate and beet juice
- Orange, carrot, and ginger detox

For breakfast, enjoy an antioxidant smoothie:

- Almond banana bread
- Honey mint
- Smoothie verde

And one of the delicious, healthy porridge options:

- Cinnamon porridge
- Berry and seed porridge
- Essential seed porridge

After breakfast, give yourself 10 to 15 minutes for a brisk walk, easy dance workout, or other gentle workout you can do in or around your home.

Allow yourself a midmorning snack of one of the following treats:

- Quinoa cups
- Hummus with olives and carrot sticks
- Mixed nuts and seeds
- Chia yogurt custard

Lunchtime is full of a lot of opportunities. Have yourself a glass of a detoxifying fruit and vegetable juice:

- Drink your greens
- The detoxifier
- Sweet carrot

For your lunchtime meal, stick to a yummy variety of

salads:

- Chickpea and artichoke sauté
- Artichoke heart and bean salad
- Super quinoa salad
- Salmon fillet salad
- Rainbow trout salad
- Anchovy salad

Between lunch and dinner, have another snack:

- Mixed melon
- Apple and carrot slices with almond butter
- Cashew coconut cookies

After your afternoon snack, give yourself 30 to 60 minutes for a moderate workout. This could be a jog, run, or taking up a yoga class, tai chi class, or other guided program with a personal trainer. You want to stick to moderate exercise as your body is still rebuilding itself and its energy.

For dinner, enjoy any one of these delicious, light, healthy, and filling meals:

- Herb and mushroom rice casserole
- Olive basmati rice
- Rice-stuffed peppers and a salad
- Dijon salmon with wild rice and steamed veggies
- Thai-style snapper
- Carrot and lentil soup
- Potato, leek, and bean soup

With dinner, have another glass of one of the fruit and vegetable detox drinks:

- Drink your greens
- The detoxifier
- Sweet carrot

Don't forget about dessert! Treat yourself to a tasty dessert such as:

- Pain perdu
- Baked stone fruits
- Rice pudding with fresh berry topping

Remember to drink a cleansing cup of dandelion tea with raw honey and a spritz of fresh-squeezed lemon juice.

As your day comes to an end, give yourself 10 to 15 minutes to perform the Gratitude Meditation, Deep Breathing Meditation, or Mindfulness Meditation.

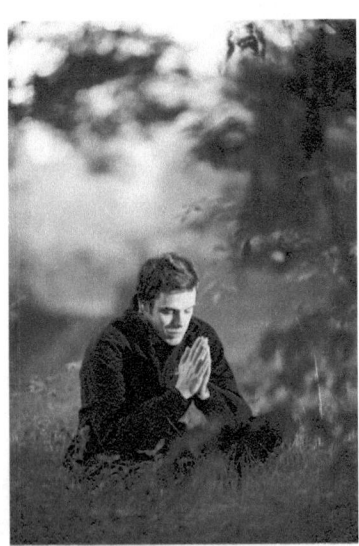

During this three-day rejuvenation period, you have more flexibility to mix and match what kinds of foods you want to eat. You can mix and match from the cleansing meals and drinks provided, as well as come up with your own. If you plan to make your own meals and follow your own recipes, be sure that they adhere to the standards of what to avoid, what to eat in moderation, and what you can eat in abundance as laid out before the seven-day flush breakdown.

Even though the three days start with 30 to 60 minutes of moderate exercise, you might still want to ease into that so you don't burn yourself out too early on. Exercise isn't just important to the cleansing, detoxing, and rejuvenating process. It is also going to help you with maintaining a healthy weight and keeping your body in an overall healthier state. Bodies that don't move and don't exercise are more prone to injury, illness, and disease, even with a healthy liver. Give yourself every advantage you can!

HOW TO USE THIS INFORMATION AND THIS PROGRAM

Use This Information for Your Own Health

Please remember that when you make changes to your diet, especially in the drastic way a flush begins, your body is going to react. It isn't going to understand why its normal routine changed so abruptly. This can cause sluggishness, fatigue, weakness, dizziness, irritability, mood swings, and a general crummy feeling.

Listen to what your body is telling you, but don't let that crumminess deter you from proceeding with the program. There is an adage that says "things have to get worse before they get better." In this case, your body has to have time to adjust to the flush before it will start benefiting from it.

That doesn't mean there isn't a little room to make allowances. If you are struggling with the exercise portion, maybe only stick to 5 or 10 minutes of exercise rather than pushing for 15 or 20 minutes. If you find that your body cannot handle the decrease in calories, give yourself leeway to eat some of the snacks provided in the Three-Day Liver Rejuvenation section for the first couple days of your flush and then taper off. These allowances will help your body adjust more smoothly to the intense detox.

If you think about it, the words detox, flush, and cleanse all imply some kind of drastic change. Change isn't always easy, and that is true for your body as well.

Detoxing regularly isn't recommended. Implementing the seven-day flush and three-day rejuvenation portion of this program isn't meant to be done every week or even every month. A cleanse paves the way for a healthier lifestyle. It is up to you to maintain your body and liver health between flushes through diet, exercise, and mindful habits.

When it comes to weight loss and maintaining a healthy weight, the easiest method for dropping weight is to eat fewer calories than you burn every day. That is why fasting is a great way to start this process. Our fasting program reduces caloric intake and promotes the burning of more calories through exercise and movement. If your body has been working hard to maintain a certain weight status that isn't your ideal weight, you might find it even more difficult to make it through the first several days of the cleanse and detox. This is because your body can almost be shocked by the rapid drop in caloric intake.

Be mindful of what your body is telling you as far as your limits. In many instances, adding in a detoxing snack that is naturally low in calories is less harmful to the flush plan than falling back to processed, unhealthy snacks to try and make yourself feel better.

A cleanse is supposed to be extreme, but it isn't meant to make you sick or hurt you in any way. In some cases, individuals with extreme circumstances might benefit from starting with the three-day rejuvenation program to ease their body into healthier foods, exercise, and lower calories before moving into the seven-day flush. If you decide to proceed in this manner to prevent your body and mind from experiencing shock, remember to still follow the seven-day flush with another rejuvenation period. You might also want to tone down the exercise portions if you don't get regular exercise.

A tip when it comes to cooking, meal prep, and fasting: If you want to save on time, you can always make a recipe that has multiple servings or double up on a recipe and then have the leftovers for lunch or dinner the next day/night. Be mindful that leftovers only keep for a few days, so you'll want to be on top of eating them or they'll go to waste.

WHEN TO DETOX: HOW OFTEN SHOULD YOU DETOX?

While there are no set "rules" on how often or how seldom you should detox, there are some health considerations. As previously stated, detoxes and flushes are not meant to be a weekly or monthly event. Several individuals find that they like to detox once a year, while others might stick to two or three times a year. Then there are some people who will do it once and be very strict in maintaining their health thereafter.

Truthfully, how often you want to detox is based on you and how you feel. The best advice we can offer is to listen to your body. You can practice that with the mindful meditations that teach you to connect with your body or by continuing to keep your liver cleanse journal after you complete the first flush.

Whenever, or if ever, you reach a point where your body feels sluggish, you feel lethargic, or those pre-cleanse symptoms begin to crop up again, that might be a good time to do another cleanse.

Even if you feel great all the time, it is impossible to keep yourself free from environmental toxins in our current society. Air pollution is one that is inescapable any time you step outside. That's not meant to discourage you from going outside because fresh air is also great for health and wellness. Environmental toxins continue to pile up in your system regardless of what lengths you take to maintain your liver health.

With that in mind, a healthy goal is to try and detox three to four times a year, every three or four months, especially if you live in a pollution-heavy environment, like major metropolitan areas or places that have suffered from oil spills or other waste disasters that have impacted the environment. Those toxic elements linger in the environment for a long time.

Now that you have completed your flush, it's time to work on maintaining the health you have just achieved.

5
HOW TO MAINTAIN A HEALTHY LIVER

Doing a liver flush and detox is a great way to establish a healthy baseline for your liver. It removes all the toxic junk that has built up in your body and gives your liver a break. The flush is just one step to long-term liver health, though. Once the liver is cleansed, if you revert to the same patterns and habits as before, that toxicity will just build right back up again.

One of the hardest parts of a healthy liver and overall health and wellness program is the maintenance. This can be difficult because maintenance is about changing your lifestyle and making conscious, daily efforts to provide support for your liver. Over time, these changes become a habit. However, in the beginning, they can be difficult, especially if they are well outside of your pre-flush lifestyle.

True lifestyle changes are a commitment. The recommendations in this chapter are going to give you a solid foundation for building habits that make and support a happy liver. At this point, you can begin to reintroduce dairy, meat, and eggs into your diet. Be mindful that in moderation, these items are fine to eat. For lifelong liver health, though, you'll want to primarily eat foods and recipes that stick to the liver health and support foods that were outlined in the previous chapter.

Diet and exercise are two of the main components of maintaining health, especially when it comes to your liver. There are other self-care practices that you can start to work into your life so that your body and mind get a chance to relax and rejuvenate between cleanses and flushes.

EXERCISE

There are so many options for exercise these days that the only real issue is finding the time. Unless you are a hardcore fitness buff, you only need 20 to 30 minutes of exercise a day to maintain yourself. While 45 to 60 minutes of exercise a day is the recommended minimum for fitness, it can be hard to find that time every day with full-time jobs, taking care of a house or a family, having pets, and other obligations.

So, when it comes to squeezing exercise in simply for the purpose of getting your body moving, 20 to 30 minutes a day can suffice. This exercise doesn't have to be incredibly rigorous either. Taking a brisk, 30-minute walk in the evening to get your heart rate up and blood flowing is a gentle exercise that keeps your body moving and helps boost your metabolism.

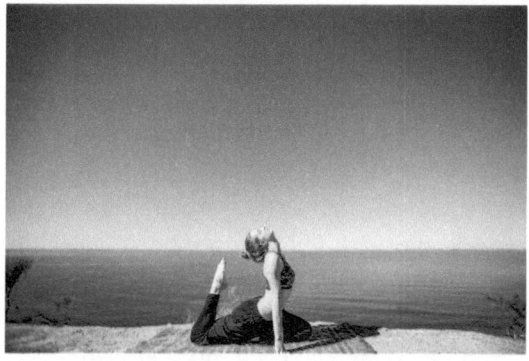

If you are crunched for time, a good tip is to look into exercise programs that you can do in your own home or around your home. A 20-minute daily jog in your neighborhood can work wonders on your body and metabolism. So can a 20-minute stretching routine right in your own living room! Between YouTube and cell phone apps, there are a lot of applications and videos you can find that instruct you in the proper way to stretch.

Through those same resources, you can find short dancing routines for fitness and programs like yoga, Pilates, and different forms of martial arts. All of these exercises can be done in your home in an open space. Just search for what you are interested in on YouTube or your smartphone app store, and you'll find a plethora of great topics and options. A lot of these services are free too!

When using apps and videos for at-home exercise instruction, look for the options that give clear and precise instructions. If a stretch isn't done correctly or a yoga position isn't held in the right way, then it can stretch the wrong muscle or not provide the benefit that it is supposed to.

Exercising at home is a wonderful way to save time and money. It does require self-management, motivation, and a willingness to learn the proper movements, holds, stretches, and muscle use so you don't inadvertently hurt yourself. There are also options for gentle and moderate exercise that you can do outside the home if you have the time and finances and feel like you would benefit more from proper instruction.

There are a lot of yoga studios around that offer different types of yoga and other kinds of exercise. You can do a quick search in your local area to find yoga, Pilates, aerobics, tai chi, aikido, martial arts, and other classes that offer different levels of exercise. You could even mix and match. Sign up for a yoga class once or twice a week, and then stick to walking or jogging the rest of the week.

Please keep in mind that if you have weight-loss goals and fitness goals, you'll want to pursue a more structured, intense workout regime. There is a difference between exercising for healthy movement and exercising for fitness.

If your goals are more oriented toward weight loss and building muscle mass, then you'll want to consider options like a gym membership. Gym memberships can be beneficial for those with tight schedules because there isn't a set time that you have to go. You can go whenever you have the time. Some gyms are even open 24 hours a day now, so if you need to go in before or after work, they will be open.

Gyms offer the advantage of other people working out, which can help motivate you to work out as well. A lot of gyms have personal trainers too. If you work with a personal trainer, they can help teach you how to move and exercise properly and help you build an exercise plan to meet your goals. A lot of gyms even have fitness classes, similar to a yoga studio, and participation is sometimes included in the gym membership fee.

There are some people who don't like exercising at gyms. Sometimes, having a gym membership seems like a good idea, and then it never gets used. Going to a gym does require motivation and self-management. Also, some people find it uncomfortable to try working out or exercising around a lot of other people, especially if some of those people are in much better shape. While it isn't a competition about being fit, this can still be difficult.

If you're the type of person who doesn't want to go to a gym, you can still find more intense workout classes or programs that have a different atmosphere. You can also develop a workout routine at home with minimal equipment, such as different weights, stretch bands with varying resistances, medicine balls, and kettlebells.

During the seven-day flush and the three-day follow-up, you were encouraged to include gentle to moderate exercise into your daily routine. That was in an attempt to keep your body active and help the detox process, but it should not have pushed you beyond the point of exertion while your body was consuming fewer calories.

When you begin forming a regular exercise regime for yourself as part of your maintenance lifestyle, you'll want to ease into the program. If you are new to regular exercise or have limited experience, start slow and gradually work up to a more difficult, longer routine. If you are an experienced exerciser but took a break during your flush, then you'll still want to ease back into your routine. Your body is in a new state of being, and it will need the time to readjust so it can handle that same level of intensity.

A few points to keep in mind while exercising:

- Ease into it
- Learn the proper way to prevent injury
- Take your time
- Find the process or method that works for you and your lifestyle
- Don't force it

- Gradually build on your stamina and fitness
- Have fun

MASSAGE AND SELF-CARE

There is more to maintaining health than just diet and exercise. Self-care is one of the least talked about methods for keeping your body and mind healthy. In a society that focuses on working harder and being more productive, concepts like taking time to relax, rejuvenate, and do self-care are simply cast aside. It is unfortunate, but you do have the ability to learn about self-care methods that can benefit you, your health, and your liver's health.

Massage

Some popular self-care activities include massage and spa services. Getting a massage isn't just lying on a table and having your sore muscles rubbed. A lot of massage therapists work to manipulate the body, removing sources of chronic pain, helping reduce tension, and correcting body posture that leads to pain and stiffness. During a massage, a lot of clients find themselves in a very relaxed state where they aren't thinking about what to make for dinner, how many emails they have to answer at work, or the like. They simply get to turn their mind off and enjoy the feeling of a healing touch.

Our society greatly underestimates the power of relaxation as a healing method. In the case of massage, while the conscious mind rests and the muscles, joints, and tissues of the body are manipulated by an outside source, the internal processes of the body have a chance to "catch up." In the case of the liver, it has the chance to kick itself into gear while the rest of the body relaxes. It can increase its own functionality during the massage.

By manipulating the muscles and joints of the body,

massage can be quite detoxifying in its own right. It can get the metabolism going and loosen up muscles and tissues that will release stored toxins, allowing them to be properly processed and eliminated. Massage has become a favorite for a lot of people, many who get massages once a month or even once a week because they get such great mental and physical benefits from it.

There are even options to get couples massages for you and your spouse or partner, or maybe you and a friend, or with a child, sibling, or parent. Couples massages end up providing a nice relaxing atmosphere for you and another person, and they aren't exclusive to romantic relationships.

Massage isn't for everyone, though. Plus, it can get pricey to have regular massages. However, there are some massage techniques that you can learn to perform on yourself at home that are especially geared toward releasing stagnant energy buildups around the liver. Since your liver is connected to several different organs and body systems, it is essentially a superhighway of energy. This self-massage technique will help keep that energy moving fluidly, thus keeping the liver functioning healthily.

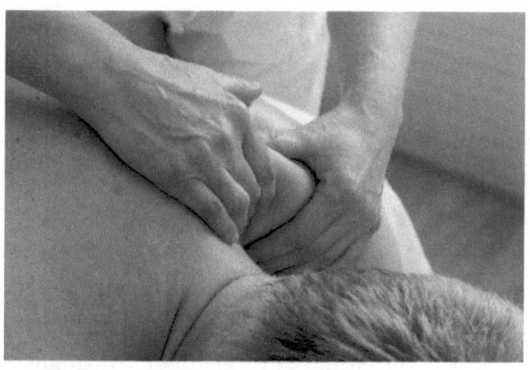

Liver Energy Stagnation Self-Massage

1. Scrunch your eyes closed tight, then open your eyes wide. Repeat 30 times.
2. On your left hand, find the point between your thumb and forefinger. It will be fleshy and a bit tender if you press down on it. Gently grasp the point between your right thumb and forefinger and perform a light, circular motion with gentle pressure on that point. Complete 30 circular motions.
3. Repeat the above step on your right hand.
4. Make a fist with your dominant hand, and starting at the base of your throat, use the ridge of your knuckles to gently tap down the center of your sternum. When you reach the bottom of the breastbone, start back at the top. Repeat this action 30 times.
5. Place the heels of your palms at the top of your abdominal muscles and with moderate to gentle pressure, sink into your muscles and push your hands down the length of your abdomen. In brushing strokes, repeat this action on the center and sides of your abdomen 30 times.
6. Locate a point directly under the nipple in the sixth intercostal area between the ribs. If you're a woman, that point will be where the underwire of your bra is or around the crease of your breast. It will be a tender divot between the ribs. Gently press on that point on both sides of the chest and do the circular massage motion 30 times. **Tip:** If you can't locate the point precisely, use the flat edge of your hand to do 30 back and forth strokes under the breast or pectoral crease to stimulate the point.
7. Repeat the abdominal massage step (Step 5).

8. Using your hand to measure the relativity for your body, hold your pointer finger, middle finger, ring finger, and pinky finger together so they are flat and level. Place the edge of your pointer finger at the base of your knee cap and use those four fingers as the measurement distance to a point on your shin. Once you have the point on your shin, trace a finger from the point to the outside of the shinbone, moving to the outside of the leg. You'll find a tender divot that is the acupressure point you are looking for. Gently massage this point in a circle 30 times.
9. Repeat on the other leg.
10. Using the same finger measurement technique, start with the protruding ankle bone on the inside of your leg. Measure along the inside leg with your fingers, and between the shinbone and calf muscle, you'll find a substantial, tender divot. Gently massage this point with a circular massage motion 30 times.
11. Repeat this step on your other leg.
12. With your pointer finger, find the point on your foot where your first and second toe bones meet. Slowly slide your finger forward until you find the soft dip between the two toes near the top of your foot. In a circular massage motion, gently massage this point 30 times.
13. Repeat the same step on the other foot.

The type of circular acupressure massage you are going to be doing is placing your thumb on the designated points and doing gentle, clockwise circles with your thumb, without removing the digit from the point.

SPA SERVICES

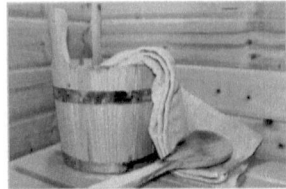

Spa services are another popular self-care practice. This doesn't just mean getting a nice manicure or pedicure. Spa services include facials; body wraps; foot, hand, and face massages; and even head massages. There can be invigorating and exfoliating scrubs as well.

Such services can get expensive; however, the techniques used are designed to be more beneficial than just clearing skin and making your hair, skin, and nails more aesthetically pleasing. Some body wraps and scrubs are designed to extract toxins from within the body. Others are designed to boost the metabolism.

Some spas have services like infrared saunas that have different sauna programs to help promote weight loss, pain relief, and detoxification. While the sauna itself doesn't make these things happen, it helps set the right wavelengths in the body so that when you stick to your exercise and diet plans, they help boost the desired outcome.

So, even though spa services are often considered a luxury for relaxation, they can be quite beneficial to the body in other ways. You might even consider making a detoxification body wrap part of your normal routine. While it won't eliminate the need for a full-body flush, it can help to stretch out the time in between cleanses and flushes.

Not to mention, spa services are usually quite relaxing and can help restore your natural energy levels. To make it even more interesting, see if you can get friends, family, or even your children to join you for a spa day. It can be a great social and bonding activity as well.

MINDFULNESS AND MEDITATION

Although the spa services above are costly, there are some self-care methods you can implement for yourself in your own home. Meditation and mindfulness practices are two very helpful self-care programs that can improve your daily life, health, and wellness.

If you are new to meditation and mindfulness, use the introductory meditations that are included in this book to help you through the seven-day flush. You can easily find phone apps, YouTube videos, CDs, and podcasts that have guided meditations, instructions on practicing meditation, and tips for mindful exercises.

Since meditation is an exercise for the mind, you'll have to ease into it, just like with body exercise. When you start, you probably won't be able to maintain the meditation for more than three to five minutes. After a while, that time will get longer. There are guided and group meditations that can last for days!

Group meditations are another way to enter the world of meditation because you can discuss your experiences with a group and talk to an instructor directly. Setting 10 to 15 minutes aside a day for meditation can drastically improve your thought patterns and lead to physical health and wellness as well as mental health and wellness.

It isn't just about learning to sit still, be quiet, and relax. There are many benefits to meditation and mindfulness practice, including benefits to your physical health and your liver function.

SELF-CARE HOBBIES

A lot of talk about self-care implies that it is intended to be some kind of self-improvement whether it be exercising, relaxing, or changing thought patterns. The essence of self-care is about making time for yourself and participating in activities that give you energy and allow you to step away from your job, your family, and your obligations and enjoy something for yourself.

Maybe you love to read, but you haven't picked up a new book in years. Start reading again. Even if just for 10 or 20 minutes a day, make it a habit and reconnect with your love of reading.

If you like playing video games, set a little bit of time aside every day to play video games. Generally, you don't want to pile on too much screen time because your eyes and brain need a break from all that blue light. However, if gaming is your passion, make time for it.

Perhaps you don't have a hobby or passion you love, but you have always wanted to learn to draw, knit, or throw horseshoes. Allow yourself the time to learn a new skill, even if that skill doesn't do anything for your job, education, or everyday life responsibilities. The point of self-care is giving yourself a break.

Even if these actions and hobbies don't specifically pertain to liver health, they do contribute to long-term mental and physical health and wellness. That long-term health and wellness does include your liver as well. So, give yourself some time and space each day for an activity you love, something you are passionate about, whatever it may be. Feed yourself and nurture yourself as an individual who isn't defined by your responsibilities. Your liver will love you for it!

DIET TIPS FOR MAINTAINING A HEALTHY AND HAPPY LIVER

Even though you have progressed beyond your seven-day flush, to maintain proper liver health and reduce toxin buildup, you are going to need to continue to be conscious about what you are eating and putting into your body. When you aren't actively detoxing, you can bring meat, eggs, and dairy back into your diet. You might decide not to, and that is completely fine as long as you are getting healthy levels of protein, minerals, vitamins, and probiotics through the rest of your diet.

Between flushes, you should consider the following tips about your diet and what is being put into your body. Not only will they help support your liver and its function, but they will help ensure that the majority of toxin buildup is from environmental influences.

HYDRATION

Fluids are one of the requirements for your body's ability to clean waste from your system. The kidneys and urinary system are waste filters, and they require fluids to process waste. Most of the substances in your body that flow and move (e.g. blood, lymph, and bile) are all fluids of some kind. So, providing your body with enough fluid to eliminate waste is important.

More than that, as your body processes waste, it loses fluids. Your body is about 60% water, so when it begins losing fluids for regular functionality, it also starts to lose water.

Staying hydrated by drinking plenty of water is going to serve your body well. It is also going to provide your liver with additional support by making the detoxing and flushing process easier as your liver processes waste.

CAFFEINE

Caffeine is one of the most overused drugs in the world. Yes, it technically is a drug. No one thinks about it in that regard, though. Coffee and tea beverages are such a normal part of daily life and society that a lot of people cannot make it through their day without multiple caffeine boosts.

The catch-22 is that relying on caffeine for energy boosts impairs the body's ability to rely on its own energy sources. Therefore, the entire body and body processes become more sluggish, especially if there isn't enough caffeine. This is one of the reasons why eliminating caffeine from the diet during a flush is so important.

When you aren't actively flushing, you should still consider moderating your caffeine consumption. In terms of helping reduce dehydration, limiting your coffee and tea intake to two cups a day, three at the absolute most, is a good idea.

Furthermore, caffeine has an incredibly long half-life, meaning it stays in the body for a long time. Sleep experts recommend not drinking any caffeinated beverages after about 11 a.m. so that the caffeine doesn't interfere with natural sleep patterns.

Sleep is another vital function for proper liver health. In fact, one of the signs of an unhappy liver is having sleep inconsistencies. Help your liver by helping your sleep and limiting your caffeine intake.

Teaching your body to function on your natural energy levels is the healthiest approach you can take. Sometimes, it can be hard to pick yourself up in the morning and get to work with a clear mind. That is why caffeine is such a coveted substance. If you can quit the habit and stick to your body's normal, natural, biological rhythm, you'll be surprised by how much better you feel over time!

AVOID ALCOHOL

Alcohol is one of the most toxic substances for the liver. It is another socially acceptable drug that is highly abused, even by people who aren't considered alcoholics. Any kind of alcohol overuse is going to put a strain on the liver.

Generally speaking, it is considered safe for women to have one alcoholic beverage a day and for men to have two alcoholic beverages a day. Now, this doesn't mean pour yourself the largest glass of wine you can and call that one drink.

By dietary guidelines, the serving size for 80-proof liquor is 1.5 ounces. A single serving size of beer is 12 ounces, and a single serving of wine is five ounces. What that means is that pouring two beers into a large glass still counts as two drinks. It also means that having a double shot of whiskey in one glass still counts as two drinks.

It is worth noting that these proportions aren't meant to be averaged over a given period. Say you drink seven beers every Saturday night, but then you don't drink any alcohol for the rest of the week. That doesn't balance out the alcohol consumption on that one night. You still greatly overtaxed your liver with those seven beers in a short period.

Drinking alcohol has become a regular, social activity. Going to a bar with friends, bar hopping, and having beer and wine at a family barbeque are considered normal. If you're serious about taking care of your liver and your long-term health, avoid alcohol when you can. Be conscious of what is considered "safe" alcohol consumption and avoid habits like binge drinking.

REDUCE UNHEALTHY FATS, PROCESSED FOODS, AND REFINED SUGARS

Grocery stores are packed with foods that are full of unhealthy fats, refined sugars, and processed foods. In fact, most commercially sold products like crackers, chips, and meat have a lot of these unhealthy additives. The downside is that consuming too many unhealthy fats and refined sugars can lead to fatty liver disease. This occurs when the liver becomes clogged with fat buildup and can no longer function as a filter.

Try sticking to leaner cuts of meat and cutting away the fat trimmings before cooking it. Meat in itself isn't necessarily unhealthy, but the excess fat can cause problems over time. You might even look at eating grass-fed, free-range, and antibiotic-free meats as well.

Processed foods are usually classified as items that come "pre-prepared." Crackers, chips, mac 'n cheese in a box, tortillas, and deli meats are examples of processed foods. They contain preservatives, and a lot of the nutritional value is stripped away during the food processing. Processed foods tend to contain hidden sugars and high levels of preservatives to extend their shelf life.

Preservatives can confuse the body into thinking that what it is eating isn't food or nutritious. Thus, the foods get processed as waste. Your body doesn't get the proper nutrients, and your liver and filtration system are working overtime every time you eat something. Those hidden sugars build up over time in a toxic way as well.

Even fruit has higher concentrations of natural sugars. Fruit intake should be limited to two or three pieces a day, and you should try to limit or cut out anything else that contains refined or added sugars. For example, store-bought peanut butter has sugar added to it, along with some unhealthy vegetable oils that translate into saturated and trans fats. You'd think peanut butter is just peanuts, but that is not how the food processing world works.

Organic, all-natural, and raw foods are becoming more widely available and more affordable. While you don't have to go to the extreme of eating organic and all-natural, you can get healthier, less processed foods from natural and organic markets, farmer's markets, and the "all-natural" food sections in your grocery store.

Eating out is another potential way to expose yourself to lots of unhealthy fats, sugars, and processed foods, especially if you're eating fast food. Sometimes, eating out is more convenient, or maybe you are craving some greasy French fries. There is no issue with that, but be mindful of how often you are eating out. Moderation is the key to preventing toxins from building up in your system. Let your body rest between your "eat outs" and give your liver ample time to clean up before eating out again. If possible, limit your eating out to once or twice a week.

The recipes in this book are all made from raw, whole food ingredients. If you get in the habit of making most of your meals in that way, you are already cutting way back on hidden sugars, unhealthy fats, and preservatives. There will be plenty of additional recipe ideas in the final chapter of this book to help get you started on filling your kitchen with foods, snacks, and meals that will benefit your liver and help reduce toxin buildup.

AVOID PARACETAMOL

Paracetamol is a common painkiller that some people use every day. The liver is the primary organ for processing and filtering drugs. Not all drugs and medications are directly hard on the liver. However, paracetamol is a liver-hitting drug. If it is taken long term, it can cause liver damage.

As a general rule of thumb, taking no more than four grams a day (about eight tablets or capsules) for no more than three consecutive days is considered safe. If you are experiencing enough pain to require more doses or long-term use, check with your doctor about alternatives. While long-term medication use will always take its toll on the body and the liver, this particular medication is harsh for the liver to process. Avoid it when you can, or ask your doctor for alternatives.

6

CAN I LOSE WEIGHT WITH A LIVER CLEANSE PROGRAM?

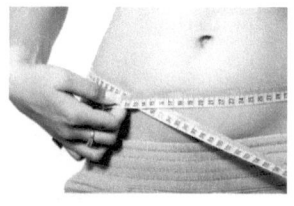

One of the most popular questions asked about liver detox programs is, can they help someone lose weight? Weight loss is one of the most common reasons why anyone might want to consider doing a program like a liver detox. It is true that a lot of people struggle to lose weight without struggling to gain it. It is also true that a liver detox program can assist in weight loss.

As a natural filter for the body, it makes sense that the liver can help to eliminate excess waste that might otherwise build up in the form of adipose tissue, or fat tissue, in the body. Because our program puts an emphasis on movement and exercise along with improving liver function and reducing toxins in the body, it can help you lose weight. The kicker is that you need to understand how weight loss occurs. With that information, you can better understand why a liver detox program can help with weight loss and how to use it to your advantage to reach your weight-loss goals.

Before getting too involved in liver detox and weight loss, let's look at some of the common misconceptions of weight loss and see why they are misconceptions.

DEBUNKING THE WEIGHT-LOSS MYTHS

It is difficult to find reliable information about weight loss and diet these days. Everyone has a new weight-loss pill, a new "proven" diet, or a revolutionary way to drop pounds in just a few days. With that much information and that many recommendations flying around, how can you determine what is true and what works?

Getting back to the basics, if we look at weight loss in terms of diet and break it down into scientific facts, we should be able to cut through some of the myths.

CALORIES

One of the most common misconceptions about weight loss is about counting calories. This myth has done more damage to weight-loss programs and regimes than any other cutting-edge, newfangled diets.

Now, a calorie is just an energy measurement. Each calorie contains 4,184 Joules of energy. This energy is what makes the body work as a complex biochemical machine.

Technically, the body is nothing more than a machine, a supercomputer if you will, that completes biochemical processes and runs off of calories. Every time you blink, raise your arm, speak, form a thought, or express an emotion, your body is transforming energy into movement or chemical processes to result in the desired outcome. The body doesn't just make its own energy, though. In the same way that a light needs a source of electricity to turn on or a computer needs a battery or cord to plug into, the body needs an energy source.

For the human body, that energy is calories. Calories come from the food we eat and the beverages we drink. On that basis, it seems like the body should be able to self-regulate. Feeling hungry when calories are running low, then feeling full when calories are fueled up. As the calories burn, that hunger feeling comes back, almost like a car's tank of gas. When the tank gets low, you fill it up. Then it runs smoothly until the fuel is burned up and the tank needs to be refilled. Your car is never "overfull" of gasoline. How, then, does the body become "overfull" of calories, leading to weight gain?

Somewhere out there is the notion that 100 calories of spinach are equal to 100 calories of Oreo cookies. While the calorie quantity is the same, the way these foods are processed in the body is not. Different kinds of sugars are metabolized by the body in different ways. While some sugars are transformed into energy, others might be processed insufficiently, causing the calorie energy to be lost as excess heat.

The different kinds of food that you eat can impact the way your body feels hunger. The brain and endocrine system produce hormones that control hunger and eating habits. If you are eating foods with micronutrients that stimulate the production of the hunger hormone, your body will feel hungry, encouraging you to eat more, even if you have consumed more calories than your body needs in a day.

Generally speaking, it is considered healthy for women to consume between 1,600 and 2,400 calories a day. For adult men, the healthy caloric intake is between 2,000 and 3,000. These numbers are where the concept of "counting calories" as a way to lose weight comes in.

Unfortunately, it is more complicated than just counting calories. Not only are different foods processed differently in the body, as discussed above, but different bodies require different caloric sustenance. For instance, if you run five miles a day and are an adult woman, you might consume more calories a day. To maintain such an active lifestyle and keep your muscle tone adequate so you don't injure yourself or end up struggling with malnutrition, you have to replenish those large quantities of calories being burned.

On the flip side, if you work at a desk 60 hours a week and the most exercise you get is walking to and from your car to your office or house, then it is unlikely that you are burning very many calories a day outside the minimum movement for calorie burning.

Exercise is only one factor to consider when calories are involved. An individual who weighs more can burn more calories running one mile than an individual who weighs less. So, weight in itself is also a consideration in how many calories are being burned in correlation to how active you are.

Another factor behind calorie burning is genetics. There are some genetic predispositions that are going to contribute to whether or not your body can keep up with burning the calories that are consumed.

Considering the metabolic pathways, how different foods are processed, and the level of exercise and current weight, you can see that there are a lot of ways calories can be processed and burned. This means that not all calories are created equal, so to speak. Thus, simply counting calories isn't going to be enough to lose weight.

Another important note about calories and counting calories. It isn't just about the kinds of sugars and foods that you are eating. It is also about what is in those foods. For example, highly processed foods and foods with preservatives are much harder for the body to digest and break down into nutrients. This is often a result of the ingredients and compounds not being naturally recognized as "food" or "nutrients" by the body. As a result, preservative-heavy foods can cause other problems that lead to weight gain.

Foods that take longer to process and digest can lead to the body feeling hungrier because nutrients haven't been processed and absorbed. You might end up eating more because the digestive system is confused about what it is trying to break down. Additionally, if the digestive system doesn't know how to process certain preservative-heavy foods, then instead of translating the foods into nutrients and caloric energy, they might get processed as waste. If large quantities of food are being processed as waste, the liver and other filtration systems can get backed up, and that waste builds up as body fat. This also means that you might be counting calories religiously, but if you're still eating junk foods and highly processed foods, you won't see an improvement in weight loss.

Once that system is backed up, it can't catch up if the same quality and quantities of food are being consumed regularly. It just adds to the problem. Going back to hunger and the body being a machine, when excess weight begins accumulating in the body, it becomes a less energy-efficient machine. What that means is more energy is required to run the machine.

Consider this: Eating 500 calories of a food like ice cream, cookies, or cake might be very easy. These are high-calorie foods. Trying to eat 500 calories of spinach, carrots, or bananas would become much more difficult. This is a great example of how different foods impact the weight-loss process. Eating 500 calories of cake is easy and probably wouldn't leave you feeling full. In contrast, you might have to force yourself to eat 500 calories of carrots, and you'd be too full to finish.

As for a body, people with excess body weight tend to eat larger portions or feel hungry more often. This is because the body needs more energy to maintain its larger mass. This is another reason losing weight can be difficult because the urge to eat more is a result of gaining weight and also hinders weight loss.

EXERCISE

Another myth about losing weight is that diet is enough. There are plenty of diet programs out there advertising low calories, low carbs, no added sugar, and so many other enticing ideas that delve into the science about how counting carbs can help lose weight. Unfortunately, a lot of those programs gloss over one major flaw. Diet alone isn't enough.

The only real equation you have to understand when it comes to weight loss is that if you consistently burn more calories than you eat, you'll lose weight. When you eat less and burn more, your body begins to burn away excess stores in the form of adipose tissue and body fat to make up for the lower number of consumed calories.

To continue to maintain your nutritional needs (not venturing into unhealthy eating habits that could lead to eating disorders) while also burning enough calories to begin dropping weight, increase your amount of exercise.

The term exercise often comes with the stigma of long workouts, heavy sweating, and being in a gym lifting weights. The beauty of exercise, though, is that movement is essentially exercise. If you are committed to losing weight, you might have to look at more rigorous exercise plans. However, depending on the amount you want to lose, or if you are just looking to maintain your weight, you don't need to go the whole nine yards.

There are plenty of light and moderate workout options that, when combined with healthier eating and liver detoxing, can assist in the weight-loss process. Exercise is about more than just burning calories, though. Exercise stimulates your metabolism. This means that your digestive system is working more efficiently. It also helps to eliminate toxins from your body that might be hindering fat burning.

It is important to acknowledge that, while the liver detox and seven-day flush can set your body up to begin losing weight, it is just one step of the process. This is why our seven-day cleanse program includes gentle exercise. Not only is it going to initiate weight loss during the flush, but it is also going to help you to get into the routine of gentle to moderate exercise.

Our goal is to give you what you need for success with your liver, long-term health, and weight-loss goals. That is why we've dedicated an entire chapter to weight loss through the liver detox program.

Another aspect of exercise you might notice is that, if you are actively losing weight, you might steadily have to increase the length of time or intensity that you are exercising for. As you lose weight, your body is going to need more exercise to burn more calories. Once you hit a target weight, you can drop back down to maintaining that weight with moderate or gentle exercise if that is your desire.

The myth about exercise and weight loss is that it isn't necessary for weight loss. Truthfully, exercise is incredibly necessary for weight loss. Both exercise and diet play important roles in weight loss and maintaining weight. What it comes down to is balancing diet and exercise.

One note about weight loss to consider is that sometimes as you exercise, you might lose body mass and adipose tissue, but you might not necessarily see a huge drop in weight. One of the reasons this can happen is that muscle tissue is denser than adipose tissue. As you lose adipose tissue and gain muscle mass, the trade-off might not equal out to a huge drop in weight. If you are experiencing this phenomenon, consider tracking muscle tone development as well as shrinking body mass in areas that were noticeably riddled with adipose tissue.

LOW-CARB VS. HIGH-PROTEIN VS. LOW-FAT DIETS

Some of the most common weight-loss diets that are all the rage include high-protein diets, low-fat diets, and low-carb diets. Each of these diets has different reasons for why they are advertised as being successful.

Taking a look at the high-protein diet, it is often advertised as increasing the body's metabolism. This is the myth of the protein diet. Honestly, the reason the high-protein diet can work is that it shrinks the appetite. Protein is a filling micronutrient, considered the most filling. When you increase your protein intake, you feel less hungry; thus, you consume fewer calories throughout the day.

One of the upsides to a high-protein diet includes losing weight without counting calories. By increasing your protein intake, you are putting fat loss on autopilot. Studies have shown that people who increased their protein consumption to 30% of their daily calories began to unconsciously eat over 400 fewer calories a day and lost as much as 11 pounds in 12 weeks (Gunnars, 2018, para 35).

Protein requires the body to use more energy to metabolize it. Thus, the high-protein diets burn fat because they use up more calories just to be processed in the body.

For almost 20 years, there have been discrepancies between the low-carb and low-fat diets. Getting down to the nitty-gritty, low-carb diets do lead to a lower caloric intake than a low-fat diet. It has been revealed through consistent testing that low-carb diets can increase weight loss two to three times more than low-fat diets (Gunnars, 2018, para 48).

As a general rule, low-carb diets lessen overall appetite. As with the high-protein diet, a decreased appetite leads to a decreased caloric intake. The low-fat diet doesn't have the same benefit. Low-carb diets also tend to drop water weight and reduce bloating in the body. This leads to a noticeable difference in weight loss as well.

Eating a low-carb diet usually results in higher protein consumption as well. Therefore, the high-protein diet benefits work in conjunction with the low-carb benefits.

If you've had any questions or concerns about calories, exercise, and the different weight-loss diets out there, hopefully, those questions have been answered. Using the information above, the next section will discuss how our liver detox program helps with weight loss.

HOW THE LIVER DETOX PROGRAM WILL HELP YOU LOSE WEIGHT

Considering the information above, one of the components of the seven-day liver flush is sticking to a low-calorie diet. Not only is your caloric intake lower since fasting is a component, but the foods you are eating are also all whole, raw foods. That means they aren't very processed and aren't high in preservatives.

Those combined qualities mean that your body will have greater ease digesting them and also in transforming them into nutrients and energy. Fewer fats, sugars, and processed chemicals will build up in your system as toxins left over from improperly digested food.

Additionally, a fasting plan, along with the low-calorie nature of the flush, will help reduce water weight in your body. Any additional bloating or excess water will be used up and eliminated. A rather large number of individuals live in an almost constant state of bloating. This is often due to an overconsumption of processed grains and dairy. There are foods that increase excess water and encourage the body to hold onto it.

By following the seven-day liver detox, you greatly cut down on water weight, which can result in noticeable weight loss. It is good to eliminate that water weight, and as a result, you can feel lighter, have more energy, and feel more physically fit.

One of the signs of a sluggish liver is unexpected weight gain. The liver can also get clogged with bad fats consumed through food. As such, it can't filter fats out of the body properly. This leads to unexpected weight gain. By completing a liver detox, you rid your body of toxins and those fat buildups. This gives your liver the chance to begin running at full speed again.

When the liver is running at full speed, it can help maintain the balance between calorie processing and weight gain. It also supports the digestive system to keep moving foods through the process of being broken down and can help filter out the waste that comes in less healthy foods.

By following the maintenance guidelines for long-term liver health, you establish a healthy system in your body that allows your liver to better maintain the desired weight in between cleanses. More than that, a healthy liver will prevent unexpected weight gain. Seeing as that is a sign of an unhealthy liver, it stands to reason that the opposite is true of a healthy liver.

Keeping in mind that a diet plan isn't enough to encourage significant weight loss, remember that a good detox program encourages an exercise routine so that it can maximize weight loss and weight management.

DETOX PROGRAMS AID IN PHYSICAL MOVEMENT IMPROVEMENT AND PHYSICAL STRENGTH

As a biochemical machine, the body requires a certain amount of lubrication to function. Think of an engine needing oil or gears needing to be greased to keep turning. There are some systems in the body that don't have an organ like the heart to pump the necessary fluids through the body. The lymphatic system is one such system. Lymph also contributes to a healthy immune system and aids in waste elimination.

When the body is filled with toxins, it becomes sluggish. This sluggishness can also manifest as stiff joints. Sodium builds up, fat builds up, and bloating and swelling can occur when the liver isn't functioning properly or if it is slow and blocked. Those buildups result in sluggishness and lethargy.

These buildups can also cause an overall crummy feeling. When you feel that sluggish and lethargic, it is difficult to have the energy or motivation to exercise. Toxins in the body can cause a lot of various problems, including difficulty with movement.

Since a detox program removes toxin buildup from the body, it also increases your energy reserves so you can take a walk, go for a jog, or go to the gym and have better movement.

Flushes and detoxes also help to improve strength and muscle tone. As you detox, you lose adipose tissue. Your body becomes leaner and more energetic. When you begin to exercise more, your leaner body will build strength and muscle faster. The more your physical shape improves, the easier it will be to maintain your desired weight.

7

BONUS CHAPTER: HEALTHY RECIPES FOR THE WHOLE FAMILY

Bonus Chapter: Healthy Recipes for the Whole Family

In this chapter, you'll find recipes for all the drinks, meals, and snacks that were referenced in the seven-day flush and three-day rejuvenation meal plans. There will be additional recipes that weren't mentioned in that chapter for you to play around with and have enough options to start with.

You'll also find the instructions for the guided meditations that were discussed in that chapter. If you can, begin making meditation and mindfulness a regular practice, even in between your liver detoxes. It can greatly impact your overall health and wellness and keep the body's energetic channels open. The self-massage technique for liver function can be amplified with regular meditation.

Detoxify Beverages Recipes

Lemona

Prep Time: 10 min
Cook Time: 10 min
Total Time: 20 min
Yields: 1 serving

Ingredients:

- 5 whole lemons
- ½ cup honey
- 3 mint bunches
- Crushed ice

Instructions:

1. Remove skins and seeds from lemons. Cut them into quarters.
2. Remove mint leaves from stems.
3. Put lemon quarters, mint leaves, honey, and crushed ice in a blender. Blitz together until well blended. Add crushed ice as needed to make a thick, frozen drink.
4. Garnish with fresh mint leaves and round lemon slices if desired.
5. Drink chilled.

Cucumber-Mint Detox

Prep Time: 10 min
Cook Time: 10 min
Total Time: 20 min
Yields: 1 serving

Ingredients:

- 10 mint leaves
- 1 cucumber

- Lemon rings and additional mint leaves for garnish (optional)
- Ice cubes
- Ice water
- 2 tbsp lemon juice

Instructions:

1. Peel your cucumber and chop it into small chunks.
2. Toss cucumber chunks, one cup of ice water, and mint leaves into your blender.
3. Blend these ingredients and then strain the pulp away.
4. Stir in lemon juice, using the blender for an even mix if desired. If needed, dilute with a little more water.
5. Pour over ice and garnish with lemon ring slices and mint leaves.
6. Drink chilled.

Pomegranate and Beet Juice

Prep Time: 5 min
Cook Time: 10 min
Total Time: 15 min
Yields: 2 servings
Ingredients:

- ½ cup beetroot, chopped
- 1 leaf of aloe vera, fresh
- 2 cups pomegranate juice
- ¼ tsp black pepper, powder

Instructions:

1. With a sharp paring knife, carefully peel away the rind of the aloe leaf. Next, peel back the yellow layer under the rind. Once the rind and yellow layer are discarded, you should have about two tablespoons of aloe vera gel. **Tip:** Skin the leaf rind the same way you'd cut the skin off a fish fillet.
2. Clean the aloe vera gel before using to get rid of any remaining rind pieces.
3. Put pomegranate juice and chopped beetroot in a blender. Blend until smooth and mixed.
4. Add in aloe gel and give it another good spin in the blender.
5. Sprinkle the black pepper on top and mix with a spoon. Transfer to drinking cups and serve immediately.

Orange, Carrot, and Ginger Detox

Prep Time: 5 min
Cook Time: 10 min
Total Time: 15 min
Yields: 2 servings
Ingredients:

- 2 oranges
- 1 carrot, large
- ½ lemon, juiced
- ½-inch fresh ginger root, crushed
- ½-inch raw turmeric root, crushed

Instructions:

1. Juice carrot and orange separately. Then add both juices to your blender.

2. Add crushed ginger root and crushed turmeric root.
3. Blend consistently for about 30 seconds.
4. Squeeze juice of half a lemon into the mix. Mix with a spoon.
5. Strain the pulp out and serve.

Dandelion Tea

Prep Time: 5 min
Cook Time: 15 min
Total Time: 20 min
Yields: 1 serving
Ingredients:

- 1 dandelion tea bag
- ½ tbsp raw honey
- 1 lemon wedge, juiced (optional)
- Boiling water

Instructions:

1. Bring about 8 oz of water to a boil in a saucepan or tea kettle.
2. While the water is boiling, put the teabag and raw honey in a heatproof mug.
3. Pour the boiling water over the teabag and honey. Stir until the honey is dissolved and then cover the mug with a plate for 2 to 5 minutes.
4. After the tea is steeped, remove the plate and teabag. Squeeze in fresh lemon juice (if desired) and give it another stir.
5. Wait until the tea is cool enough to drink. Enjoy it warm.

ANTIOXIDANT SMOOTHIES

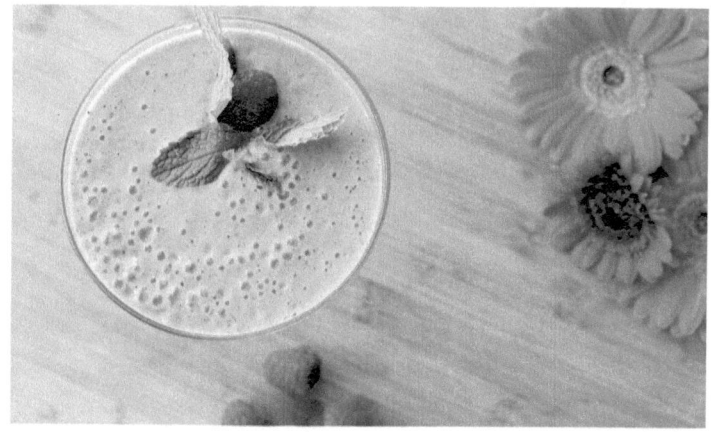

Almond Banana Bread

Prep Time: 5 min
Cook Time: 5 min
Total Time: 10 min
Yields: 2 servings
Ingredients:

- 2 bananas, peeled
- 1 cup almond milk
- 3 tbsp walnuts (more for optional garnish)
- 3 tbsp rolled oats
- 1 ½ oz baby spinach
- 1 tsp cinnamon (more for optional garnish)
- 1 cup ice

Instructions:

1. Combine all non-garnish ingredients in a blender and blitz until smooth and creamy.
2. Transfer to drinking glasses and garnish with a sprinkle of walnuts and cinnamon.
3. Enjoy immediately.

Honey Mint

Prep Time: 5 min
Cook Time: 5 min
Total Time: 10 min
Yields: 2 servings
Ingredients:

- 4 oz honeydew, cubed
- 4 oz grapes, any kind
- 1 zucchini, chopped
- 1 bunch mint (save leaves for optional garnish)
- 3 tbsp cashew nuts (more for optional garnish)
- 1 cup ice
- 1 cup water

Instructions:

1. Toss all your ingredients into the blender and give it a whirl.
2. When the ingredients are blended, transfer to drinking cups. Garnish the drinks with a few cashews and mint leaves on top.
3. Serve immediately and enjoy!

Smoothie Verde

Prep Time: 5 min

Cook Time: 5 min
Total Time: 10 min
Yields: 2 servings

Ingredients:

- 1 apple, chopped
- 2 tomatillos, husked
- 1 lime, juiced (additional slices for optional garnish)
- 1 ½ oz collard greens
- 1 tbsp pea protein
- 1 cup water
- 1 cup ice

Instructions:

1. Add all the ingredients to a blender. Blend them until smooth.
2. Transfer the smoothie to drinking glasses and garnish with lime slices if desired.
3. Enjoy immediately.

FRUIT AND VEGETABLE JUICES

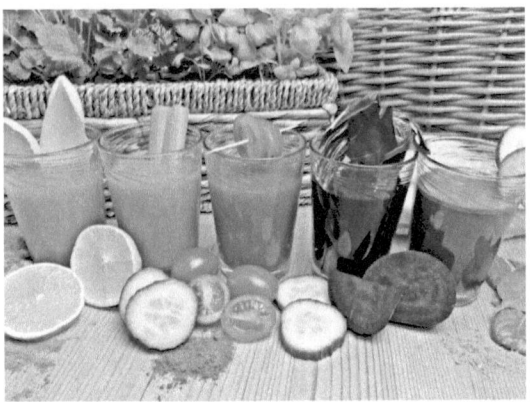

Drink Your Greens

Prep Time: 10 min
Cook Time: 5 min
Total Time: 15 min
Yields: 4 servings

Ingredients:

- 6 celery stalks, chopped
- 2 large cucumbers, peeled and chopped
- 2 medium apples, chopped
- 2 cups baby spinach leaves
- ½ lemon, peeled
- ¼ to ½ cup parsley leaves
- 1 2-inch fresh ginger root, skinned

Instructions:

1. Put the ingredients through a juicer one at a time, or blend them with a fine blender or immersion

stick blender. If you use a blender option, strain any pulp from the finished product.
2. Pour over ice to serve.
3. Enjoy immediately.

The Detoxifier

Prep Time: 10 min
Cook Time: 5 min
Total Time: 15 min
Yields: 4 servings

Ingredients:

- 6 carrots, chopped
- 3 medium-sized beets, chopped
- 2 apples, chopped
- 1 2-inch fresh ginger root, skinned
- ½ lemon, peeled

Instructions:

1. One at a time, feed your produce ingredients through a juicer. If you don't have a juicer, use a fine blender or a wand immersion blender to mix. With the blender option, you may need to strain any pulp from the juice.
2. Transfer your juice to ice-filled glasses and enjoy.

Sweet Carrot

Prep Time: 10 min
Cook Time: 5 min
Total Time: 15 min
Yields: 4 servings

Ingredients:

- 10 carrots, chopped
- ¼ cup fresh parsley leaves
- 2 apples, chopped

Instructions:

1. Use a juicer to juice your ingredients one at a time. Alternatively, you can blend your ingredients in a fine blender or with a wand immersion blender. You'll want to strain out any pulp if using the blender method.
2. Pour into glasses with ice cubes and drink immediately.

BREAKFAST

Cinnamon Porridge

Prep Time: 5 min
Cook Time: 10 min
Total Time: 15 min
Yields: 1 serving
Ingredients:

- ½ cup traditional oats
- ½ tsp ground cinnamon
- 1 cup boiling water
- Raw honey, to taste (optional)

Instructions:

1. Set the heat to high to boil water in a saucepan with a lid. Add in oats and reduce to a simmer before covering with the lid.
2. Allow oats to cook, checking their progress occasionally but not stirring.
3. Once the water has been cooked into the oats, remove from heat. Let sit for 1 to 2 minutes before transferring oats to a heatproof bowl.
4. Sprinkle cinnamon on oats and mix. Add in raw honey to taste if you want a slightly sweeter porridge.
5. When it is cool enough to eat, enjoy while warm.

Berry and Seed Porridge

Prep Time: 10 min
Cook Time: 10 min
Total Time: 20 min
Yields: 1 serving
Ingredients:

- ½ cup traditional oats
- 1 tsp essential seed mix (see recipe in Additional Recipes)
- ¼ cup mixed berries (blueberries, raspberries, blackberries)
- 1 cup water

Instructions:

1. In a saucepan with a lid, bring the water to a boil. Add in the oats and reduce to a simmer. Then put the cover on the oats.
2. Let cook until the water has cooked into the oats, checking occasionally. You don't need to stir them.

3. Remove from the heat and allow to sit covered for a few minutes. Then transfer them to a heatproof bowl.
4. Mix in your seeds and fruits. Let cool enough to safely eat and enjoy.

Essential Seed Porridge

Prep Time: 5 min
Cook Time: 10 min
Total Time: 15 min
Yields: 1 serving
Ingredients:

- ½ cup traditional oats
- 1 tsp essential seed mix (see recipe in Additional Recipes)
- 1 cup water
- Raw honey, to taste (optional)

Instructions:

1. Pour water into a saucepan that has a lid. On a high temperature, boil the water. Toss oats into the water and reduce to a simmer. Then cover with the lid.
2. While they are cooking, check on them now and then, but do not stir. When the water has cooked into the oats, remove from the heat. Keep them covered and let them sit for 1 to 2 minutes. Then transfer the oats to a heatproof bowl.
3. Mix in your essential seed blend and add a little raw honey to taste if you'd like. Allow the oats to cool a little and then enjoy them while still warm.

LUNCH/DINNER

Chickpea and Artichoke Sauté

Prep Time: 5 min
Cook Time: 5-7 min
Total Time: 13 min
Yields: 4 servings

Ingredients:

- 1 can chickpeas, rinsed
- 1 can artichoke hearts, rinsed
- 1 tbsp garlic, minced
- 2 tsp turmeric powder
- 3 tbsp extra virgin olive oil
- ½ tsp sea salt
- ½ tsp black pepper, ground
- Fresh-squeezed lemon juice

Instructions:

1. Heat a skillet over medium heat. While the pan is heating, combine the chickpeas and artichoke hearts in a bowl. Add in olive oil and seasonings. Toss until evenly coated.
2. When the pan is hot, pour in the ingredients from your bowl. Shake the pan so that nothing sticks.
3. Cook the mixture for 5 to 6 minutes, stirring every minute. Remove from heat when the chickpeas are brown.
4. Squeeze the fresh lemon juice onto your sauté and mix. Then transfer to a bowl and eat warm. You

can also chill it and eat later. It keeps for three days when refrigerated.

Artichoke Heart and Bean Salad

Prep Time: 10 min
Cook Time: 10 min
Total Time: 20 min
Yields: 1-2 servings

Ingredients:

- 3 marinated artichoke hearts
- ½ red onion, chopped
- ½ can red or black beans
- Super Salad Greens Mix (see recipe in Additional Recipes)
- 1 tbsp black olives, chopped
- 1 tbsp olive oil
- Handful of fresh basil leaves
- ½ cup cherry tomatoes, halved
- 1 garlic clove, crushed
- 1 tbsp tomato purée

Instructions:

1. Put the tomato purée, olive oil, basil leaves, and crushed garlic in a blender. Using the pulse setting, blend the ingredients into a dressing.
2. In a large bowl, mix salad greens, beans, onion, olives, artichoke hearts, and cherry tomatoes.
3. Drizzle your dressing over the tossed ingredients and serve.

Super Quinoa Salad

Prep Time: 10 min
Cook Time: 30-60 min
Total Time: 1 hour
Yields: 1-2 servings
Ingredients:

- ⅓ cup quinoa
- ⅔ cup water
- 1 tsp reduced salt vegetable bouillon powder
- ½ sweet potato, cubed
- ½ red pepper, chopped
- ¼ cup cherry tomatoes, halved
- 1 clove garlic, crushed
- t tbsp olive oil
- 2 tbsp pumpkin seeds, unsalted
- Super Salad Greens Mix (find recipe in Additional Recipes)
- Salt and pepper, to taste
- Blended olive oil and apple cider vinegar, equal parts (optional dressing)

Instructions:

1. Preheat the oven to 450 degrees.
2. Toss the sweet potato and red pepper with olive oil, garlic, and salt and pepper. Lay on a baking dish.
3. When the oven is ready, put the veggies in and roast for 30 minutes, stirring at least twice during the cooking period. If they need longer, add time in 10-minute increments.
4. While the veggies are roasting, bring some water to a boil in a saucepan and then add bouillon powder and quinoa. Stir and reduce the

temperature so it begins to simmer.
5. Put your salad greens in a large mixing bowl. Toss with the halved cherry tomatoes and the pumpkin seeds.
6. Chill your veggies and quinoa once they are done cooking. Then toss them in with the rest of the salad.
7. Enjoy as is or drizzle with a little olive oil and apple cider vinegar mix.

Salmon Fillet Salad

Prep Time: 15 min
Cook Time: 15 min
Total Time: 30 min
Yields: 1 serving
Ingredients:

- 1 small salmon fillet, skin or no skin
- Super Salad Greens Mix (find recipe in Additional Recipes)
- ⅓ cup lentils, boiled
- Salt and pepper, to taste
- Olive oil

Instructions:

1. Preheat the oven to 450 degrees. Season the salmon with olive oil, salt, and pepper. Place the salmon skin-side down (if applicable) on a nonstick baking sheet.
2. Cook in the oven for 10 to 15 minutes. Check the internal temperature of the salmon to ensure it is at 145 degrees.

3. While the salmon is cooking, boil the lentils in a saucepan over the stove.
4. When the salmon is cooked, flake it into smaller pieces with a fork. Chill the salmon and lentils.
5. Toss salmon flakes and lentils in with your salad greens and enjoy.

Rainbow Trout Salad

Prep Time: 10 min
Cook Time: 15 min
Total Time: 25 min
Yields: 1-2 servings
Ingredients:

- 1 rainbow trout
- 1 garlic clove, sliced
- Super Salad Greens Mix (see recipe in Additional Recipes)
- 1 lemon, sliced
- Olive oil
- Dash of salt
- Dash of pepper
- ½ cup cherry tomatoes, halved
- ½ cup black beans, cooked

Instructions:

1. Preheat your oven to 400 degrees. Cover a baking sheet in foil with enough tin foil to wrap around the fish.
2. Put the fish on the foil. Drizzle with olive oil, then season with salt and pepper on both sides.
3. Tuck lemon slices and garlic slices around fish.

Wrap the foil and close it around the fish in a little pocket.
4. Bake in the oven for 10 to 15 minutes. Check at 10 minutes. You'll know the fish is done when it is opaque and flakes with a fork.
5. Fillet the fish in half and fork out the cooked meat inside.
6. In a large mixing bowl, combine your greens, cherry tomatoes, and beans. Mix in the fish and you have a complete salad.

Anchovy Salad

Prep Time: 10 min
Cook Time: 10 min
Total Time: 20 min
Yields: 1 serving

Ingredients:

- 4 to 5 anchovies, sliced
- Super Salad Greens Mix (see recipe in Additional Recipes)
- ¼ cup black olives, chopped
- ¼ cup cherry tomatoes, halved
- Equal parts olive oil and apple cider vinegar, blended (optional dressing)

Instructions:

1. In a large mixing bowl, toss your greens, olives, tomatoes, and anchovies. Drizzle with the optional dressing if desired and enjoy!

Herb and Mushroom Rice Casserole

Prep Time: 5 min
Cook Time: 35 min
Total Time: 40 min
Yields: 3 servings

Ingredients:

- 2 cups cooked brown rice
- 1 ½ cups vegetable stock/broth
- 4 cups mushrooms, chopped (portobello, oyster, trumpet)
- 5 green onions, chopped (use white and green parts)
- 2 bunches fresh dill, stems removed and minced
- 1 bunch fresh parsley, stems removed and minced
- 1 tsp garlic, minced
- 1 tsp dried oregano
- ½ tsp cayenne pepper
- ½ tsp black pepper, ground
- 2 tbsp olive oil

Instructions:

1. Preheat the oven to 350 degrees.
2. Warm your skillet on medium heat and then add the olive oil, letting it heat in the skillet. Cook the garlic and onion together, mixing regularly, until onions are translucent, about 5 minutes.
3. Stir in the cayenne, oregano, and black pepper. Mix and cook for one minute.
4. Add in the mushrooms, dill, and parsley. Stir and cook until the mushrooms are soft, usually around 5 to 10 minutes, then remove from the heat.
5. In a casserole dish, combine the rice with the

mushroom mixture. Pour the vegetable broth over the casserole.
6. Cook in the oven uncovered for about 30 minutes. The casserole will have a brownish crust over top.

Olive Basmati Rice

Prep Time: 5 min
Cook Time: 15 min
Total Time: 20 min
Yields: 1 serving
Ingredients:

- ⅓ cup basmati rice
- ⅔ cup water
- Handful of basil leaves
- Handful of baby spinach leaves
- 1 garlic clove, crushed
- 3 tbsp olive oil
- 1 tbsp pumpkin seeds, unsalted
- 3 tbsp olives, minced
- Juice from ½ lemon
- Ground black pepper

Instructions:

1. In a saucepan, bring water to a boil and then add the basmati rice. Stir and bring down to a simmer. Put the lid on and let the rice cook.
2. In a skillet over medium heat, cook garlic, basil, and spinach in olive oil. When they are cooked, drizzle with lemon juice and season with black pepper.
3. Mix the spinach and basil mix into the cooked

rice. Then toss in the olives and pumpkin seeds, giving another good stir. Enjoy!

Rice-Stuffed Peppers and a Salad

Prep Time: 10 min
Cook Time: 75 min
Total Time: 85 min
Yields: 1-2 servings
Ingredients:

- 2 bell peppers
- ½ cup brown rice
- 1 cup water
- 4 mushrooms, chopped
- 2 tbsp pine nuts
- 1 clove garlic, minced
- 3 tbsp olive oil
- Sea salt and black pepper, to taste
- 1 (8 oz) can tomato paste
- Salad

Instructions:

1. Preheat the oven to 350 degrees.
2. Boil one cup of water in a saucepan. Add in brown rice and stir. Reduce to a simmer, then cover and let cook until done, about 20 minutes.
3. In a skillet, warm the olive oil on medium heat. Add in the garlic and let cook until browned. Then toss in mushrooms and sprinkle in the salt and pepper to your liking.
4. Cook the mushrooms until soft, about 5 to 10 minutes. Then remove from the heat.

5. While the rice and mushrooms are cooking, cut the tops off your bell peppers. Remove the stems, seeds, and membranes, leaving a hollowed-out shell. Set them on a flat or shallow baking dish, open end up.
6. Mix your mushrooms and rice and add in the pine nuts and tomato paste. Stir all ingredients.
7. Portion the rice mix into the bell peppers.
8. Cook in the oven uncovered for an hour.
9. Serve the peppers warm with a green salad on the side.

Dijon Salmon With Wild Rice and Steamed Veggies

Prep Time: 10 min
Cook Time: 30 min
Total Time: 40 min
Yields: 1 serving
Ingredients:

- 1 small salmon fillet, skinned
- Dijon mustard
- Himalayan pink salt
- Ground black pepper
- 1 cup veggies (broccoli, green beans, carrots, or a combo)
- ¼ cup wild rice
- ½ cup water
- Olive oil

Instructions:

1. Preheat the oven to 450 degrees.
2. Set the salmon fillet on a nonstick baking sheet.

Drizzle with a little olive oil. Then smother with Dijon mustard and season with Himalayan salt and black pepper.

3. Bring water to a boil in a saucepan. Add in the wild rice and stir. Reduce the rice to a simmer and cover. Allow to cook for about 20 minutes.
4. Put the salmon in the oven. Cook for 10 to 12 minutes.
5. Put the veggies in a medium-sized saucepan with a half-inch to an inch of water on the bottom. Cover partway and bring to medium-high heat, using the steam to cook the veggies. Don't cook them too long if you like them to have a little crunch.
6. Check the fish to make sure it has an internal temperature of 145 degrees.
7. Serve the salmon over a bed of wild rice and with a side of steamed veggies.

Thai-Style Snapper

Prep Time: 10 min
Cook Time: 8-10 min
Total Time: 20 min
Yields: 4 servings
Ingredients:

- 8 shallots, minced
- 1 ½ lb red snapper, washed, patted dry, cut into 2 pieces
- 2 tbsp minced garlic
- 2 tbsp fresh ginger, minced
- ½ teaspoon sea salt flakes
- 2 limes, halved
- 2 tbsp peanut oil

- 1 red chili, dried and crumbled
- 2 tsp turmeric powder
- 1 cup brown rice, cooked

Instructions:

1. Toss the fish in the turmeric powder and let sit.
2. Use a mortar and pestle to grind half the sea salt and the shallots into a paste. Transfer to a mixing bowl.
3. Using the mortar again, grind the rest of the sea salt with the ginger and garlic.
4. Over medium heat, warm a large skillet. Add ½ tablespoon of the peanut oil and the shallot paste to the warmed skillet.
5. Cook for 5 minutes until brown. Add in the ginger and garlic mix along with the crumbled chili and cook for another 5 minutes.
6. Put the remaining oil in the skillet and put in the two fish pieces. Cook for about 5 minutes. Then flip.
7. Cook the flipped fish for about another 2 minutes. Check to make sure it is done and properly flaky, then remove from the heat.
8. Squeeze the lime halves over the fish and serve over a bed of brown rice.

Carrot and Lentil Soup

Prep Time: 10 min
Cook Time: 10-15 min
Total Time: 25 min
Yields: 2 servings
Ingredients:

- 2 carrots, chopped
- ½ cup split red lentils, cooked
- ½ yellow onion, chopped
- 2 cups vegetable stock
- 1 celery stick
- Super Salad Greens Mix (see recipe in Additional Recipes)
- 1 garlic clove, crushed
- ½ tbsp olive oil
- Salt and pepper (optional)

Instructions:

1. In a large pot, add the vegetable stock, carrots, celery, onion, garlic, lentils, and olive oil.
2. Raise the soup to a boil. Then lower the temperature and allow to simmer. Allow to simmer for 10 minutes, stirring occasionally.
3. Stir in the salad greens and cook for another 2 to 3 minutes. Enjoy warm. Season with salt and pepper if you want more flavor.

Potato, Leek, and Bean Soup

Prep Time: 10 min
Cook Time: 15-20 min
Total Time: 30 min
Yields: 2 servings
Ingredients:

- 2 potatoes, cubed
- 2 leeks, sliced
- 1 cup cannellini beans, cooked
- 2 ½ cups water

- 3 tsp vegetable bouillon powder
- 1 tsp olive oil
- 2 garlic cloves, crushed
- Ground black pepper

Instructions:

1. Stir the vegetable bouillon powder into the water in a large pot. Add in the potatoes, leeks, olive oil, garlic, beans, and black pepper.
2. Bring the entire pot to a boil, stirring regularly. Reduce to a simmer and stir occasionally. Allow to simmer for 15 minutes, then enjoy!

Snacks
Quinoa Cups
Prep Time: 5-7 min
Cook Time: 20 min
Total Time: 25 min
Yields: 24 mini muffins
Ingredients:

- 1 cup quinoa, cooked
- ½ cup zucchini, shredded
- ½ cup sun-dried tomatoes, finely chopped
- 2 large eggs
- 1 egg white
- 2 tbsp green onion, chopped
- 2 tbsp fresh parsley, chopped
- 1 tbsp fresh basil, chopped
- Sea salt
- Black pepper, ground

Instructions:

1. Set your oven to 350 degrees.
2. Add all the ingredients in an appropriately sized mixing bowl, and use salt and pepper to season.
3. Using a mini muffin pan, grease the pan with cooking spray or olive oil.
4. Evenly spoon the mixture into the muffin pan, filling each cup about ⅔ of the way.
5. Bake for 15 to 20 minutes until they are golden brown on the outside. (If you only have a regular-sized muffin pan, grease it up and fill the cups ⅔ of the way. Set timer for 25 to 30 minutes and allow cups to bake.)
6. Cool for 10 minutes before removing them from the pan. Use a paring knife to gently pull them from the pan.
7. Enjoy warm or cooled.

Hummus With Olives and Carrot Sticks

Prep Time: 5 min
Cook Time: 5 min
Total Time: 10 min
Yields: 3-5 servings
Ingredients:

- Container of hummus
- Can of black olives
- Jar of kalamata olives
- 4-5 carrots

Instructions:

1. Open your hummus and transfer the amount you

want to eat into a small dish or keep it in the resealable container it comes in.
2. Wash and peel the carrots. Cut the carrots in half. Cut those halves into quarters, the long way, to make carrot sticks.
3. Strain the olives.
4. Arrange all the carrots, olives, and hummus on a plate for yourself or a platter to share. Dip olives and carrots into hummus.

Chia Yogurt Custard

Prep Time: 5-10 min
Total Time: 5-10 min
Yields: 2 servings
Ingredients:

- 1 cup coconut or almond milk yogurt
- ¾ cup coconut milk or almond milk
- ¼ cup orange juice
- 6 tbsp chia seeds
- 2 tbsp raw honey
- ½ tsp vanilla extract
- ½ tsp cinnamon
- ½ tsp sumac, ground

Instructions:

1. Pulse the chia seeds, sumac, and cinnamon in a blender. Make a coarse powder.
2. Add the milk, yogurt, honey, and orange juice. Then pulse with the chia seed powder. It should become the same consistency as thick soup.

3. Allow the custard to set in the fridge overnight or for at least an hour before enjoying.
4. You can top with some nuts or berries to make it more interesting.

Mixed Melon

Prep Time: 10 min
Total Time: 10 min
Yields: 2-3 servings

Ingredients:

- Honeydew
- Cantaloupe
- Watermelon
- Muskmelon

Instructions:

1. Cut each of your melons in half. Keep one half and put the other away to use for something different.
2. Cut each of your melon halves into quarters. Use a sharp, long knife to carefully remove the rinds.
3. Cut the rindless melon slices into smaller cubes, about ½ inch in size.
4. Mix all the melon pieces in a large bowl for a nice variety.
5. Store in the refrigerator and enjoy as a snack for up to three days.

Apple and Carrot Slices With Almond Butter

Prep Time: 10 min
Total Time: 10 min
Yields: 2-3 servings

Ingredients:

- Almond butter
- 1 large apple
- 2 carrots

Instructions:

1. Wash and peel the carrots. Wash and core the apple.
2. With a sharp paring knife, cut the apple into six to eight slices.
3. Cut the carrots in half. Then cut those halves into quarters, the long way, to make carrot sticks.
4. Dish some almond butter into a bowl or cup.
5. Dip carrots and apple slices into almond butter and enjoy!

Cashew Coconut Cookies

Prep Time: 5-10 min
Cook Time: 20-25 min
Total Time: 35 min
Yields: 24 small cookies
Ingredients:

- ¾ cup almond flour
- ½ cup cashew nuts, finely ground
- ½ cup coconut oil
- ½ cup raw honey
- 1 cup shredded coconut, unsweetened
- 1 cup traditional rolled oats
- ½ cup coconut milk
- 1 tbsp lecithin

- ½ tsp salt

Instructions:

1. Begin by preheating your oven to 350 degrees.
2. Combine the honey, ground cashews, ½ cup almond flour, coconut oil, and lecithin. Cream these ingredients together in a blender or with an immersion wand blender.
3. Add in the remaining almond flour, shredded coconut, oats, and salt. Use a spoon to mix with the cream to combine evenly.
4. Pour the milk in and stir until the mixture is smooth.
5. Line a baking sheet with parchment paper. Using two spoons, gather some dough between the spoons and drop it on the parchment paper, leaving about two inches between each cookie.
6. Bake cookies 20 to 25 minutes. Check near the end for doneness. You'll want to remove them from the oven while still a little soft as they will harden while they cool.
7. Let cool and enjoy!

Desserts
Pain Perdu
Prep Time: 10 min
Cook Time: 15-17 min
Total Time: 25 min
Yields: 6 servings
Ingredients:

- 1 loaf of bread, sliced
- ½ cup almonds, slivered

- 1 ½ cup almond milk or coconut milk
- 6 eggs
- 4 tbsp raw honey
- 2 tsp salt
- 1 tsp orange zest
- 1 ½ tsp vanilla extract
- 1 tbsp butter

Instructions:

1. Using a large mixing bowl and a whisk, whisk together the milk, eggs, vanilla extract, honey, orange zest, and salt.
2. Preheat a large skillet on the stove over medium heat.
3. Place the bread slices in a shallow dish or plate with a lip.
4. Pour the whisked mixture over the bread slices. Let them soak for 2 minutes and then flip them over, letting them soak for another 2 minutes.
5. Pour the almonds into a shallow dish or bowl. Dip one side of each bread slice into the almonds to give each slice one side of an almond coating.
6. Melt the butter in the pan. Working in batches, add slices of bread to the pan. Let them sauté for 3 minutes and then flip, sautéing for another 3 minutes. They will be golden brown when done.
7. An optional topping is fresh berries and a little maple syrup.

Baked Stone Fruits

Prep Time: 10 min
Cook Time: 15 min

Total Time: 25 min
Yields: 4 servings
Ingredients:

- 2 plums, pitted and cut into slices
- 2 peaches, pitted and cut into slices
- 2 apricots, pitted and cut into slices
- 2 nectarines, pitted and cut into slices
- ½ cup apple juice
- 2 tbsp raw honey
- 2 tbsp butter, unsalted and cut into small, cold cubes

Instructions:

1. Preheat the oven to 400 degrees.
2. In a four-by-six casserole dish, alternate fruit slice layers until the dish is filled.
3. Top the fruit with the butter cubes and then drizzle honey over the fruit and butter.
4. Pour apple juice over everything and let soak until the oven is ready.
5. Bake for about 15 minutes or until there is a light char on the outer rim of the fruit slices.
6. Turn off the heat, but let the fruit sit in the oven for an additional 5 minutes.
7. Remove the dish from the oven. Leave it to sit and cool for 10 minutes before eating.

Rice Pudding With Fresh Berry Topping

Prep Time: 10 min
Cook Time: 35 min
Total Time: 45 min

Yields: 4 servings

Ingredients:

- 2 ½ cups coconut or almond milk
- ⅓ cup white rice, uncooked
- 1 egg
- ¼ cup brown sugar (can use sugar substitute like honey or maple syrup, liquid measurements differ from solid)
- ¼ tsp cinnamon
- 1 tsp vanilla extract
- ⅓ cup mixed berries or chopped fruit
- Pinch of salt

Instructions:

1. In a saucepan, bring the milk to a boil and then add the rice and salt. Bring back to a boil and stir. Then reduce to a simmer and cover with a lid. Cook until tender, about 20 minutes.
2. In a mixing bowl, whisk the egg and brown sugar. Add half of the milky rice to the egg mix and stir.
3. Add the sugar and rice mix back to the saucepan with the rest of the rice. Keep on low heat and cook while continually stirring for 5 to 10 minutes until pudding thickens. Be careful not to boil.
4. Remove from heat and stir in the vanilla extract and cinnamon.
5. Chill pudding and then top with fruit or berry topping and enjoy.

ADDITIONAL RECIPES

Super Salad Greens Mix

Prep Time: 10 min
Total Time: 10 min
Yields: 1 serving
Ingredients:

- ¼ bag baby spinach leaves
- ¼ bag watercress
- Handful of basil leaves
- Handful of parsley leaves
- 1 tbsp extra virgin olive oil
- Spritz of lemon juice

Instructions:

1. Rinse and dry the greens and herbs. Chop the leaves and herbs, but not finely.
2. Toss in a mixing bowl with the lemon juice and olive oil. Use it as a salad green base.

Mixed Nuts and Seeds

Prep Time: 5 min
Total Time: 5 min
Yields: 5-6 servings
Ingredients:

- ¼ cup almonds
- ¼ cup walnuts
- ¼ cup cashews
- 2 tbsp chia seeds
- 2 tbsp flax seeds
- 2 tbsp pumpkin seeds, unsalted

Instructions:

1. Combine nuts and seeds in a bowl. Toss or use a spoon to mix them evenly.
2. Store in a glass jar with a sealable lid. One handful is a serving size.

Essential Seed Mix

Prep Time: 5 min
Total Time: 5 min
Yields: 5-6 servings

Ingredients:

- Flax seeds
- Chia seeds
- Sesame seeds
- Sunflower seeds, unsalted and without a shell
- Pumpkin seeds, unsalted

Instructions:

1. In a pint-sized mason jar, fill the jar halfway with equal parts of flax seeds, sesame seeds, and chia seeds. Fill the other half of the jar with equal parts sunflower and pumpkin seeds.
2. Leave about ¼ to ½ inch of free space at the top. Screw the jar lid on and shake to mix the seeds.
3. Store in the glass jar in the fridge or in a dark pantry to avoid direct sunlight.
4. Use in porridges, as a snack, and in other seed recipes.

8

BONUS CHAPTER: GUIDED MEDITATIONS

When meditating, it is recommended that you set yourself up in a quiet, relaxing setting in a room or space that won't be disturbed where you can be alone. You might even find that it is helpful to dim the lights, put on some relaxing music, and light some candles or some incense.

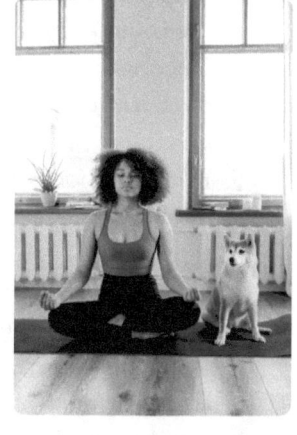

Sometimes after a meditation, you may feel lightheaded or dizzy. If you do experience that kind of sensation, place your palms and forehead on the floor to ground yourself. Then drink a glass of cold water. Take it easy getting up and moving around.

Even after your seven-day cleanse and three-day rejuvenation, try making meditation a regular part of your routine. This will continue to aid your mental and emotional health, which, in turn, helps to reduce toxin buildup in the body.

GRATITUDE MEDITATION

1. Sit or lie down comfortably in a chair, on a couch, or in your bed. Start with a series of deep, steady breaths, relaxing your body into heaviness and your mind into thoughtlessness.
2. Let yourself go; let your mind go; let your body go; drift away from yourself.
3. Slowly bring your hands together. Put your palms together, fingers pointing to the ceiling in the prayer position.
4. Position them so they are hovering over your heart but not touching your body.
5. Take a nice deep breath in and hold your breath to the count of four. Then slowly release that breath. Once again, take a deep breath in. Hold here to the count of four before gently releasing your breath.
6. Bring your focus to the tips of your pointer fingers by gently pressing your fingertips together on your forefingers.
7. As you apply pressure to your fingertips, say "I have love," and then release the pressure.
8. Press your fingertips together again and say "I have trust," before releasing the pressure.
9. Go ahead and push the tips of your pointer fingers together, saying "I have faith," and then relax your finger muscles.
10. Engage your muscles, pressing your pointer fingers together, and say "I have courage." Release the pressure on your fingers.
11. Once more, apply pressure to your forefingers, pressing the tips together, and say "I have

gratitude." Release the pressure and take a deep breath in and a slow breath out.
12. Begin to come back to your body, reconnecting with yourself and your physical surroundings. Open your eyes and ground yourself if necessary.

DEEP BREATHING MEDITATION

1. Find a space and time where you can be alone. Make sure you will be undisturbed for the duration of this meditation. Sit or lie down comfortably on a bed or chair. Close your eyes.
2. Take some deep, calming breaths, soothing your mind and body. Let go of the physical world around you. Drift away from yourself.
3. Begin to focus on the way that you breathe, taking a long, heavy inhale through your nose while counting to three. When your lungs are inflated, pause and hold your breath to the count of three. As you exhale, release slowly, counting all the way up to six.
4. Breathe in again while counting slowly up to three. Hold for another three seconds. Slowly exhale all the way up to six.
5. Continue this breathing pattern for 20 full breaths. Inhale, hold, and exhale.
6. When you have finished your breaths, gently become aware of yourself again. Open your eyes and ground yourself if you need to.

MINDFULNESS MEDITATION

1. Find a time and place where you can be alone

without interruption. Sit or lie down on a bed or chair. Close your eyes.
2. Start with some deep, relaxing breaths. In through the nose, then out through the mouth. Relax your mind and body.
3. In through the nose and out through the mouth.
4. Continue this breathing pattern, becoming more aware of your breaths and how your breathing feels.
5. On your next full breath, inhale and exhale. Complete the cycle by counting to the number "one." With your next full breath cycle, count to the number "two."
6. Keep counting your breaths, focusing on the inhale through the nose and the exhale through the mouth, all the way up to 10.
7. Naturally let your breathing shift back to a regular pattern. Slowly come to your physical body and look around, opening your eyes. Ground yourself if you feel the need.

GETTING THE WHOLE FAMILY INVOLVED

If you have children or a significant other or spouse who you live with, consider getting them involved in keeping their livers healthy as well. Some good ways to get everyone involved include:

- Family meal planning
- Cooking meals as a family
- Eating family meals without distractions (like smartphones, television, and reading materials)
- Making goals and plans with your family and

helping keep each other on task (e.g. exercise or weight-loss goals)
- Setting aside some "family time" or relaxing days where the whole family can spend time together doing something fun (it doesn't have to be elaborate)

There are plenty of ways to make liver health as well as long-term health and wellness interesting for the whole family. Come up with your own list of ideas to get everyone involved.

EPILOGUE

At the beginning of this book, you were promised a liver detox program that would help you lose weight, detoxify your body, and support long-term liver health as well as overall health and wellness.

Through the seven-day liver flush program and the three-day rejuvenation plan, you can achieve those goals when you make the commitment to stick to the plan. You have everything you need to foster a healthy liver and lifestyle through diet as well as through meditation and exercise. These key points to the reading are what are going to guide you toward your success.

From here, you should start planning your liver detox flush. It is recommended that you get a notebook to begin keeping track of how you feel and how your body changes. Some people find it helpful to begin taking daily selfies so they can compare how they look at the beginning of the program and track the subtle changes they might not otherwise notice.

Another good idea for preparing for your fasting cleanse is to stock your kitchen and refrigerator with the items that you'll be using for your fast week and three-day rejuvenation period. Having as much of that stuff ready will help to reduce and eliminate impulse purchases during your cleanse that can pull you away from the overall goal.

Please remember that this program does require some commitment and motivation. You'll have to manage yourself, which is another way a journal can become a helpful tool to keep yourself on track. If you have a spouse or significant other, consider getting them involved so they can also help you reach your goals. Liver detoxification is about your health, short and long term.

It is never too early to consider preventatives for future toxin buildups. It is also possible to successfully reduce, repair, and halt liver damage that has already occurred. Give your liver a fighting chance! This program is all about you and your liver. You can make the most of it for yourself.

Be mindful of the fact that what you've learned in this book isn't a substitute for medical care, treatment, or advice. It is still advised that you discuss a liver detox program with your primary care physician, especially if you have a preexisting condition.

If you found the information in this book helpful, we encourage you to leave a review. Reviews are greatly appreciated, and they help other people like you find this information to benefit themselves. Thank you, and good luck with your liver!

DISCUSSION SECTION
A SUCCESS STORY FOR INSPIRATION

Kelly had struggled with Epstein-Barr, a fatty liver, adrenal fatigue syndrome, and thyroid issues for years. She also had eczema and achy joints. No amount of medications or treatment were able to resolve all of her issues. Then, she discovered a liver cleanse program that changed her life.

For a month, Kelly stuck to her cleanse diet. She followed all the dietary restrictions that were outlined in the seven-day liver detox plan. At first, she felt a lot of mixed feelings. She struggled with insomnia, blood sugar fluctuations, headaches, soreness throughout her body, and flu-like symptoms.

As she moved into week two of the cleanse, her blood sugar began to regulate. She had strange dreams, but she was at least sleeping better. Her eczema began to fade, but she started to break out on her face.

Week three gave way to a drastic decrease in rosacea, eczema, and joint pain. Her mental clarity was improved, and she started feeling more energetic. She also had more-regulated blood sugar. By the time she made it to week four, the only adverse symptom she had was vertigo. Everything else had cleared itself up, and she was feeling so much better physically and emotionally.

In her one-month plan, she lost about 20 pounds and her skin and joint conditions cleared themselves up completely! Kelly is a success story when it comes to the benefits and outcomes of a liver cleanse and detox. She stuck to her plan, and even two years later, she still has been able to keep the weight off and stay in optimal health and shape. Kelly's success can be your success too!

REFERENCES

AAC. (2020, March 3). *Vitamin K deficiency.* https://labtestsonline.org/conditions/vitamin-k-deficiency#:~:text=The%20signs%20and%20symptoms%20associated,and%20injection%20or%20surgical%20osites

Baur, E. (n.d.). *Rice pudding.* Simply recipes. https://www.simplyrecipes.com/recipes/rice_pudding/

Beer, C. (2016, September 12). *Benefits of liver detoxing.* mitoQ. https://www.mitoq.com/blog/blog/benefits-of-liver-detoxing

Cottis, H. (n.d.). *My weight loss story.* Whole lifestyle nutrition. https://wholelifestylenutrition.com/health/my-weight-loss-story/

Crichton-Stuart, C. (2018, March 14). *What are the symptoms of low vitamin E.* Medical news today. https://www.medicalnewstoday.com/articles/321800

Dr. Lu's Nourishing Life. (2018, March 21). *Liver energy stagnation self massage.* Youtube. https://www.youtube.com/watch?v=kqOQzy-hFRI

Editorial Staff. (2019, February 21). *Flush away fat and feel your energy soar with a 'liver reboot' detox diet.* Woman's world.

https://www.womansworld.com/posts/diets/liver-detox-diet-165783

Editorial Staff. (2020, May 8). *How much alcohol is safe to drink daily?* Alcohol.org. https://www.alcohol.org/faq/safe-level-of-drinking/

Felman, A. (2018, February 22). *Why do signs and symptoms matter?* Medical news today. https://www.medicalnewstoday.com/articles/161858#:~:text=Share%20on%20Pinterest%20A%20sign,is%20who%20observes%20the%20effect.

Greenblender. (2020). *5 antioxidant-powered smoothie recipes.* https://greenblender.com/smoothies/8428/antioxidant-powered-smoothie-recipes

Gunnars, K. (2018, May 8). *6 reasons why a calorie is not a calorie.* Healthline. https://www.healthline.com/nutrition/6-reasons-why-a-calorie-is-not-a-calorie

Healio Hepatology. (2016, October 28). *Depression, anxiety prevalent in young people with liver disease.* https://www.healio.com/news/hepatology/20161028/depression-anxiety-prevalent-in-young-people-with-liver-disease

Hoffman, M. (n.d.). *Picture of the thyroid.* WebMD. https://www.webmd.com/women/picture-of-the-thyroid#1

Huang, X. Liu, X. Yu, Y. (2017, May 8). *Depression and chronic liver diseases: Are there shared underlying mechanisms.* US national library of medicine. https://www.ncbi.nlm.nih.gov/pmc/articles/PMC5420567/

Johnson, Larry E. (2019, August). *Vitamin A deficiency.* Merck manual. https://www.merckmanuals.com/professional/nutritional-disorders/vitamin-deficiency,-dependency,-and-toxicity/vitamin-a-deficiency#:~:text=Vitamin%20A%20deficiency%20can%20result,and%20low%20vitamin%20A%20levels.

Kalra, A. Yetiskul, E. Wehrle, C. J. Tuma, F. (2020, May 24). *Physiology, liver.* NCBI. https://www.ncbi.nlm.nih.gov/books/NBK535438/

Kunces, L. (2018, August 29). *Do I need a liver detox?* Thorne. https://www.thorne.com/take-5-daily/article/do-i-need-a-liver-detox

Modern Honey. (2018, September 18). *Healthy juice recipes.* https://www.modernhoney.com/healthy-juice-cleanse-recipes/

Nall, R. (2018, April 2). *What does the liver do?* Healthline. https://www.healthline.com/health/what-does-the-liver-do

NCBI. (1989). *Diet and health: Implications of reducing chronic disease risk.* https://www.ncbi.nlm.nih.gov/books/NBK218749/#:~:text=Vitamins%20A%2C%20D%2C%20E%2C,similar%20to%20that%20of%20fats.

Patrick. (2016, January 27). *The one-week detox diet.* Patrick Holford. https://www.patrickholford.com/advice/the-one-week-detox-diet

Physiol J. C. (2007, November). *Liver regeneration.* US national library of medicine. https://www.ncbi.nlm.nih.gov/pmc/articles/PMC2701258/

Prima Team. (2015, May 2). *The liver cleanse diet: Nine days to a healthier you.* https://www.prima.co.uk/diet-and-health/healthy-living/news/a21940/liver-detox-diet/

Sengupta, S. (2020, April 21). *11 delicious detox drink recipes.* NDTV food. https://food.ndtv.com/lists/10-delicious-detox-drink-recipes-1684332

Verde Valley Naturopathic Medicine. (2019, March 1). *Benefits of a liver cleanse.* http://vvnaturopathic.com/blog/2019/1/18/benefits-of-a-liver-cleanse

Vere, C. C. Streba C. T. Streba L. M. Ionescu, A. G. Sima, F. (2009, June 28). *Psychosocial stress and liver disease status.* US national library of medicine. https://www.ncbi.nlm.nih.gov/pmc/articles/PMC2702105/

Whitcomb, I. (n.d.). *Diet for cirrhosis: My 3-day healing meal plan for liver disease.* further food. https://www.furtherfood.com/3-day-meal-plan-my-cirrhosis-liver-disease-healing-diet/

Woreta, T. A. (2020). *Detoxing your liver: Fact versus fiction.*

Johns Hopkins Medicine. https://www.hopkinsmedicine.org/health/wellness-and-prevention/detoxing-your-liver-fact-versus-fiction

WebMD. (n.d.). *Can a detox or cleanse help your liver?* https://www.webmd.com/digestive-disorders/liver-detox#1

WebMD. (n.d.). *Vitamin D deficiency.* *https://www.webmd.com/diet/guide/vitamin-d-deficiency#1*

All images sourced from https://pixabay.com/

7 STEP GUIDE TO FLUSH TOXINS AND RESTORE LIVER HEALTH

THE CELERY JUICE CLEANSE

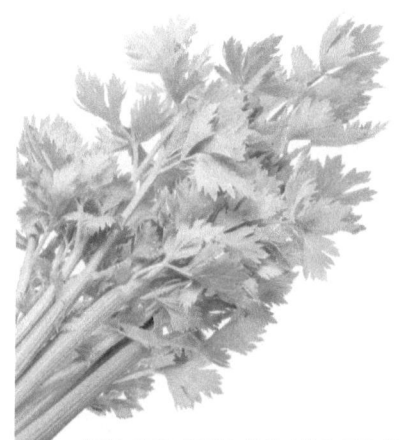

RESET YOUR BODY

RELIEF FOR BRAIN FOG, ACNE, ECZEMA, ADHD, THYROID DISORDERS, DIABETES, SIBO, ACID REFLUX AND LYME DISEASE

GABRIELLE TOWNSEND

INTRODUCTION

> If you don't take care of this the most magnificent machine that you will ever be given...where are you going to live?
>
> — KARYN CALABRESE

Congratulations on purchasing *The Celery Juice Cleanse Hack,* and thank you for doing so. Are you ready to feel better and improve your mind, body, and spirit? If so, keep reading. What you choose to eat has a lifetime effect on your body, mood, and physical health. Your diet may help prevent some chronic diseases and speed up your recovery time after accidents. We will go over how you can change your lifestyle, what you should eat, and other ways to get the maximum benefits of juicing. Bad gut health has been shown to influence your moods, your energy level, and how you feel in general. This book will cover the benefits of using celery juice to detox, improve your gut health, and have more energy.

Juicing can change your life as it has changed many others. You will learn about the myths and misconceptions about celery juice. We will work together to change the way

INTRODUCTION

you think about juicing and food nutrition. You may be asking yourself, why drink celery juice instead of just eating it? Juicing provides all the benefits of eating celery and more. It separates the juice from the ribs in the stalk that tend to get stuck in your teeth and cause annoyance. In addition to separating the ribs from the stem, it is easier to digest and detoxify your body. We will also cover seven steps to help make juicing part of your daily life and exactly what a juice cleanse is. I look forward to helping you change your life with juicing like it has many others.

There are plenty of books on this subject on the market, thanks again for choosing this one! Every effort was made to ensure it is full of as much useful information as possible. Please enjoy! Now let's head to the store!

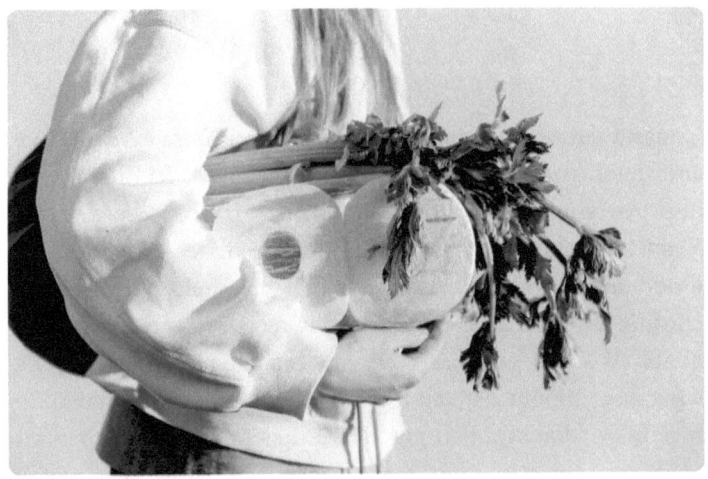

1

WHAT IS THE CELERY JUICE CLEANSE?

WHY CELERY JUICE CLEANSING IS SO POPULAR

A juice cleanse is a healthy way to detox your body. The way juicing works is using a juicer to squeeze the fresh juice from the fruit or vegetable, separating the liquid from the pulp. Fruits and Vegetables are essential to your health. Fruits are high in vitamins, minerals and are anti-inflammatory. Trying to make sure you eat the right amount of vegetables day to day can be a difficult, if not impossible, task. When juicing is part of your daily life, you get all of the vitamins and minerals in one drink.

Americans are always in a hurry. Most of the time, it's easier to stop at Mcdonald's to grab a breakfast sandwich on your way to work. After a full day at work and the errands after work, it is easier to grab a pizza for dinner. Another thing many of us enjoy doing is having a nice relaxing dinner eating out. It solves the hassle of cleaning up after eating and allows you to have a much-needed break. When we aren't grabbing take-out or eating out, Our dinner may consist of boxed or frozen dinners filled with additives, high sodium, added sugars, and fat. These dinners don't taste as good as fresh food, and they make our liver work harder to break the food down. Juicing helps the liver to detox and recover from this type of diet. Foods that are high in fat or loaded with chemicals slow down your liver's ability to break down foods as efficiently as it needs to. A juice cleanse can help your liver have time to detox and rest so that it can work its best.

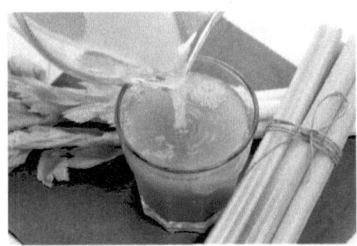

Your gut has such an influence on your body, from your mood to your day-to-day energy. Everything you eat is broken down in there. Digestive systems contain healthy bacteria and immune cells that help to fight off infections and viruses. Another job of the intestines is to communicate with the brain. The brain is what decreases the risks of depression and gives you energy. Giving your gut time to detox and rest is an essential part of your overall health.

The liver's primary function is to filter the blood from the digestive tract before it goes to the rest of your body. Your liver also filters and detoxifies chemicals and drugs. The drugs that it detoxifies can be prescription, illegal, or vitamins, and your liver does not know the difference. A juice cleanse gives you the vitamins and minerals you need therefore lowering the number of vitamins you take. The anti-inflammatory properties found in celery juice may limit the amount of medication you take to get the same benefits.

When you eat, your liver has to break down the food to get the nutrients. Your body then sends the nutrients to all the cells to energize your body. When you are juicing, it extracts those vitamins, so your body doesn't have to. Doing this gives you more energy.

If your goal is to lose weight juicing can help with that. The juice helps you feel full for a more extended amount of time, therefore, decreasing the amount of food you consume. The toxins being flushed from your body also aids in weight loss. Some of the weight loss, in the beginning, will come from water weight, but in changing the way you eat and your relationship with food, you will lose fat instead of water weight. One key in juicing is changing the way you eat. While juicing, you consume less fat, decreasing your cholesterol and therefore decreasing your heart disease or stroke risk.

Juicing also helps your skin look fresher and clearer. Your body no longer has to break down all of your food. Instead, the juice goes straight to your cells. You will look healthier, feel better, and get a glow that wasn't there before. Juicing is excellent when you are sick; it breaks down the juice for you. It keeps your immune system healthy to prevent sickness. A healthy immune system can also help with chronic conditions like allergies.

Juicing can also help you sleep better. Eliminating coffee and alcohol from your diet enables you to go to sleep more comfortably and sleep longer. Juicing increases your fiber intake, which is one of the keys to better sleep. You haven't been eating junk food all day, and this helps your sleep cycle improve. After reading so much about the celery juice cleanse and how it has helped countless people feel better and increase their energy, you may want to give it a try but wonder where to start. It's a straightforward program. Just start adding it to your morning routine—each morning, when you get up, drink a glass of celery juice. Typically you should drink 16oz, but you can start with less and work your way up.

The first and most important thing is to drink the juice

every morning for a month. Drinking it daily helps you get the maximum benefits and gives you time to see how you feel. Another thing you must remember it does not add anything to your juice. In order to get the full benefits, the juice needs to be free of any additives. Daily, people are coming up with ideas to add this or that to the juice cleanse, but that will defeat the purpose of giving your liver a chance to reset. Even if you add protein powder, thinking it will help, it will dilute the juice. Some people who start this cleanse wonder what is the difference if I throw the celery in with my morning smoothie? There is a big difference. Juicing is when you extract the water and nutrients from the fruits or vegetables, and smoothies blend the whole fruit and vegetable skin. The fiber that is in the stalk needs to be removed to get the benefits of celery.

What do you do in the morning when you get up? Do you, like so many, start brewing coffee or drink a glass of water first? The good news is you can keep that glass of water then wait 20 minutes or so to drink your celery juice. While you wait, you can start juicing the celery. In about as much time as it takes to start your coffee, you can have the juice ready.

Once you drink the juice, you need to wait another 20-30 minutes to eat breakfast. Eat something simple, a smoothie, some fruit, or oatmeal. It is vital to make the oatmeal with water and not milk. One of your goals with the celery cleanse is to detox your liver. Staying away from fats is essential while you are doing the cleanse.

If you eat fats while doing the juice cleanse, it causes the liver to break down the food instead of giving it time to heal. Not only does eating foods high in fat cause your liver to start working it will also dilute the celery juice. Diluting the juice is something you want to avoid. We want your liver to relax for a month and let the celery juice do its job. Some examples of the fats to avoid are Avocados, all dairy, eggs, and cooking oils. The good news about this is you can eat healthy carbs.

When you think of the celery juice cleanse, you probably think of Anthony William (the Medical Medium). The Medical Medium published a book in 2015 about celery juice's celery juice's healing benefits ad caught on like wildfire. Many people have become a fan of him due to his holistic approach. If you look on Instagram, you will notice he has 1.6 million loyal followers.

On Instagram, look at the Medical Mediums before and after pictures of what celery juice has done for people. It's no wonder this detox has caught on. From clearer skin to a healthier digestive tract, it appears that a lot of people have a positive experience in using the juice and what it does for them. Word of mouth is one of the best ways to tell people about a new product working for you, and this also helped celery juice gain its popularity.

Markets started to see the sales of celery going up, at times making it difficult to keep it in stock. Markets also see an increase in sales whenever medical reports indicate a product has health benefits or a celebrity or scientific claim. Now, if you search online for celery juice, you will see over 56 million results.

To further increase its popularity, celebrities' such as Sylvester Stallone, Liv Tyler, and Gwyneth Paltrow say how much the celery juice has benefited them. Stars are looked up to, and once they endorse something, others are bound to try it. Juicing continues to gain popularity as more people try it and share all the benefits. Today, many say the celery juice diet craze is a global movement and believes it is here to stay.

In an interview with the Washington Magazine, Gwyneth Paltrow said she does not need to cleanse at all. In the article,

Paltrow also adds, the only time she does a cleanse is if she's doing it for her website; otherwise, only a yearly cleanse. Surprisingly, an article in her magazine, Goop, written in 2016, about the benefits Anthony Williams is said to be one of the most unconventional yet insightful healers today.

❦ 2 ❦

THE BENEFITS OF CELERY JUICE
THE REASON THIS CLEANSE MUST BE A MAINSTAY IN YOUR DIET

Celery has not been studied as much as other vegetables, so we are just discovering the benefits of this vegetable. Most people do not know there is a difference between celery and celery juice. At the same time, both have health benefits; they are not all of the same benefits. Celery stalks have fiber, where celery juice does not. During the juicing process, the celery is pressed instead of chopped so that you get pure juice.

While celery and celery juice have similar benefits juicing gives you benefits that eating it whole does not. When you juice the celery, it removes the pulp and cuts out fiber. In removing the fiber, your body can break it down and digest it. Without the liver has to work to break it down, it can detox.

I realize that we talk a lot about how amazing celery juice benefits your liver, and there is much more to learn about that hard-working organ. Juicing has numerous healing effects on your liver due to all the nutrients and antioxidants. When your liver becomes bogged down with many fats and foods filled with chemicals and hard metals, it causes it to be sluggish and unable to filter as usual.

While reading this, you will read a lot about the Epstein-Barr virus (EBV). I want to give you a bit of information about this virus to know what it means when you hear it. EBV is a member of the herpes virus family, and this is one of the most common human viruses in the world. Most people will get some form of this at some point in their lives. One way to prevent this is drinking plenty of fluids to stay hydrated and get plenty of rest. You will read many ways that celery juice helps both of these. Celery juice is very hydrating and helps you go to sleep and stay asleep longer.

The endocrine system consists of glands that produce and secrete hormones vital for many of our bodies' functions. Some of the tasks that the endocrine system supports are respiration, metabolism, reproduction, sensory perception, movement, sexual development, and growth. An underactive endocrine system's symptoms include fatigue, depression, anxiety, craziness, weight gain, hair loss, and infertility. Hormones can overproduce or under-produce; both of these are harmful to our bodies.

Juicing offers support to the endocrine system by the easily digestible nutrients that are in a concentrated form. Increasing juicing helps improve fertility and ease the symptoms of premenstrual syndrome. I'm going to mention the liver again. It is also responsible for helping to regulate and breaking down hormones and eliminating them. Celery helps to support the liver so it can bind and excrete hormones to keep balance.

This herb contains plant hormones that help to rejuvenate the endocrine system. Your thyroid is part of the endocrine system, and as we age, it gets a bit bogged down at doing its job. Celery juice helps to kick start the thyroid and bring it back to working as it should. The endocrine system helps heal many autoimmune disorders, and celery juice helps reset the endocrine system to fight against the pathogen's attack.

Sodium cluster salts, unlike table salt, this type of salt benefits your body. The cluster salts remove the toxic salts that you have been adding to your food for years. When you have blood tests done, they may pick up the added sodium. The tests do not know the difference between healthy and unhealthy sodium. It is also possible to pick up the sodium that breaks down in your body due to the flush.

During a celery juice cleanse, you are replacing high sugar drinks with healthier options. It's interesting to note that drinks like soda, coffee, energy drinks, and specialty coffees increase our sugar intake by 50% and add 500 extra calories. Celery is antioxidant-rich. It has been shown that eating food high in antioxidants can lower the risk of chronic ailments, such as heart disease and diabetes.

Drinking as little as 250mg of celery juice three times a day is enough to keep your blood sugar at an average level. For people who have diabetes, built-up fat causes a lot of inflammation in the body that can cause kidney complications; celery juice reduces inflammation. Celery's antioxidants properties can help to reduce inflammation. While celery juice might not cure diabetes, it can help keep your blood sugar under control and help relieve symptoms. Another interesting fact is that in September 2015, a study conducted showed that the flavonoid luteolin, a nutrient in celery, might help in diabetic neuropathy or nerve damage.

Some have said that drinking celery juice every day has helped them recover from addictions. One of the causes of addiction is EBV, which is caused by the build-up of hard metals in your body. When you go through detox, your body dehydrates. Celery is made of water and keeps you hydrated. Our brain and liver go through a lot of damage during drug or alcohol addiction. Celery juice helps to reverse that due to the healing properties contained in the juice. Experts believe that many addicts are insulin resistant. Celery has a very low glycemic index which helps to even out blood sugar.

Strep, sinusitis, and strep are common symptoms of EBV in early life; this could contribute to acne. Typically, you will be prescribed antibiotics to help fight the infection when you have one of these illnesses. Medical research and science are under the misconception that acne is due to hormones. The excess oils found on skin that's thought to cause acne are sebum oil trying to fight the strep bacteria. The clusters of sodium salts found in celery help break up the strep, while the vitamin C in the juice clears up the acne.

I don't know if you have ever had to deal with a sinus infection, but they are awful. Your ears hurt, your nose hurts, your face hurts, your whole body hurts from sinuses. Some people who have chronic sinusitis opt for surgery to see if it can fix the problem. The surgery does help for a short time, and then they come back, and it can be worse than before. Drinking celery juice long-term can help with sinus issues. The sinuses are ties to the lymphatic system, and celery juice quickly reaches the sinus cavity and boosts the body's immune system.

Arthritis is a painful and chronic disorder that is caused by inflammation in one or more joints. There are multiple types of arthritis-like RA (Rheumatoid Arthritis), PsA (Psoriatic Arthritis), and Scleroderma. Each of these is believed to be an autoimmune disorder when there are indications that it may be part of the Epstein-Barr Virus. The Epstein-Barr Virus causes inflammation in joints and nerves. We already know that celery juice is full of anti-inflammatory properties, so drinking it makes sense.

The liver is one of the only organs of the body that can heal itself. When it gets overrun with toxins, you will notice you become sluggish, and so your digestive system does too.

When it stops functioning correctly, your kidneys and skin have to work harder. This more challenging work causes your skin to hold more impurities that the liver usually eliminates. Celery juice helps break down these toxins so that your liver can work more effectively, which helps to clear up your skin.

In America, 6 in 10 adults have a chronic disease, and 4 in 10 have two or more. Tobacco use, poor nutrition, lack of physical activity, and excessive alcohol use are the main risk factors of chronic diseases. Celery juice has been shown to reverse some of these effects on your body. Drinking celery juice each day helps the cravings of eating foods high in sugar, and instead, you are drinking juice full of unique nutrients. The hydration and healing benefits help with the hydration and healing of your body.

Celery juice increases bile strength as a part of the process of healing the liver. Most people are not fond of the increased bile, but it fades as the liver heals. It is excellent for people who have had their gallbladder removed by helping the liver recover. Once your gallbladder is removed, it becomes more difficult to digest substances in many foods we eat daily. A robust, healthy liver is essential in helping to break down and digest these substances.

Fibromyalgia is a chronic pain syndrome caused by the brain and nerves overreacting to pain signals. The effects of it on an individual differ from person to person, the symptoms are varied, and it can take years for a diagnosis to be made. While there is no cure for fibromyalgia, there are ways to control it, many of these consist of different types of medications and a healthy diet. Celery juice is wonderful to incorporate as part of your diet, especially with its anti-inflammatory properties. While it will not help you, it may help you to get over the inflammations quicker.

This miracle juice can also help with respiratory issues like asthma and bronchitis. Determining what your asthma trigger is essential in determining the best way to handle it. Do you frequently forget your inhaler or have to search endlessly for it? If you are going on an outing with friends or family, will there be something in the air that will affect your asthma? These are typical questions that people dealing with chronic disorders need to ask themself.

There are different types of asthma, and some of them have underlying vital conditions. Epstein-Barr is a common virus that is the reason for many chronic disorders that the medical community has not been studied. Another cause could be the toxic and heavy metals that we are exposed to daily. Emotions, stress, and mood disorders can mimic the symptoms of asthma. Think about if you have ever had a panic attack. What were your symptoms? I bet there was difficulty breathing, feeling a heavy pressure on your chest, and sometimes hyperventilating like it was almost impossible to catch your breath. There are many instances where people went to the hospital thinking they were having an asthma attack or even some who believed they had a heart attack. It is easy to see why asthma can be confused by other issues that many of us suffer.

Now let's talk about mucus, its function, and how it relates to our respiratory system. Mucus is a much-needed substance. It is a protective substance that is used in a variety of areas of our body. A major component of mucus is mucin. It is located as a lubricant, barrier, or dense material, which means that mucus protects our body's surface and assists our immune systems.

What happens is when the mucus starts fighting off infection, it can trap bacteria which causes phlegm. The phlegm is responsible for respiratory issues. Asthma, bacterial and viral infections cause your airways to make too much mucus, and This is where celery juice can help. Hydration is an essential part of thinning the mucus, so it is easier to remove it from your system. We already know that celery juice has excellent detox properties that will remove the toxins and heavy metals in your body.

Unlike many herbs, there isn't a limit on how much celery you can consume. You can safely drink multiple glasses of it without the harmful side effects. It is also interesting to note the essential oil in celery juice helps with anxiety and gout. Celery can also be used as a relaxant which is a great way to relieve pressure. Gout is caused by the buildup of uric acid in the body. Celery has compounds that break up the uric acid helping the inflammation to recede and

Most of us have heard of the mid-afternoon crash when all of our energy seems to fade, and all we want is a nap or a sugary treat. Celery juice helps to keep that mid-afternoon tiredness away. With many foods, drinks, and sugary foods, a sugar spike comes after eating them, and it fades away after a short time. The benefit of celery juice is there is no spike in energy; it is a steady stream that lasts all day.

After the 30 day cleanse, should you keep drinking it? Many people do stop drinking it every morning but continue drinking it 2-3 times weekly. They want to keep the health benefits they noticed during the 30 day cleanse. Yes, the taste takes a bit of getting used to, but you start looking forward to it once you get used to it.

In continuing to make celery juice part of your daily ritual, you keep getting the day-to-day benefits, keep your gut and digestive system healthy, detox your liver and keep eliminating unhealthy heavy chemicals you ingest. Getting celery in your diet means you will get a ton of nutrients in your diet also. You will continue to keep hydrated, and replacing those high sugar drinks is not suitable for your health.

Celery helps to support digestion. Often known as the natural laxative, celery also works as a natural way to balance your pH. You don't need a lot of these enzymes to build up weakened digestive walls. In balancing the pH, it can reverse many digestive issues such as bloating, constipation, and many other stomach issues. If your stomach acids are low, this decreases your energy levels while your stomach is digesting food. If you frequently get ulcers or have acid reflux, celery increases your gastric mucus.

Other than your overall health, one of the best benefits of celery juice is the increased energy. It is a great way to wake up with energy and a good mood before a long day. There is no caffeine in the juice, so you do not have to worry about continuously drinking highly caffeinated drinks. The beta-carotene in celery juice is converted to vitamin A, which protects from cell damage, providing you with increased daily energy.

While drinking celery juice every day, even with the many benefits, is not a magic cure-all. Suppose you continue to eat unhealthy foods and continue with a high-stress life while not benefitting as much. Without combining celery juice with a healthy lifestyle, your body will have to work too hard to get all of the benefits. If you do not enjoy its taste and can't do it daily, try to work towards doing it 1-3 times a week.

The celery juice cleanse similar to any other diet change while offering the same benefits to everyone. The cleanse will affect everyone in different ways and at different times. Someone may see the benefits the next day and another person in a week. A person's eating style will have an impact on how their system detoxes. The person who does not eat much meat and instead fills up on vegetables will likely have an easier time detoxing than the person whose primary diet consists of meats, potatoes, and desserts.

❦ 3 ❦
NOTABLE TOXINS TO BE AWARE OF
FROM ALERGIES TO PESTICIDES

When people hear about something new, something that sounds too good to be true, people are understandably skeptical. Due to the lack of scientific studies on celery, there is a lot unknown about the benefits. There are many rumors and untruths out there about celery juice. In this chapter, we are going through some of the most frequent rumors and giving you the correct information. Celery is a unique Vegetable filled with so many vitamins, minerals, and healing abilities. Instead of doubtful, I want to ensure you know the full benefits of drinking it with confidence.

Many say drinking celery juice is a fad and will fade away like so many trends do. One is the amount of detox cleanses that have claimed to work wonders for your body. It makes sense that people would believe this is a fad based on the information alone. The celery juice cleanse is different because other detoxes want you to stop eating while doing the detox. We don't want you to stop eating, just make better nutritional choices and steer clear of fats.

TOXINS

There are natural toxins in every food you eat. The difference between natural toxins and harmful ones is they are natural and do not contain enough toxins to cause damage. Toxins that naturally occur in fruits and vegetables are beneficial to your health. Pink rot occasionally happens in a fungus that occurs when the celery is wilting and going bad. This fungus rarely occurs and is not toxic to humans. Still, it does lower the benefits of celery juice.

Food allergen

Some people may be allergic to celery, however very few people are allergic to celery juice. Many times what people are experiencing is the effects of the celery juice clearing out the pathogens, killing the viral bacteria are destroyed, and this releases whatever was fueling the harmful bacteria. The neurotoxins and viral waste will be going into your bloodstream for elimination which can cause the feeling of food allergies. If the celery juice triggers an instant allergic reaction, it would be because the juice instantly expelled the toxins out of our liver, or it could come from an instant shock to our system. If this is the case, change to cucumber juice and slowly incorporate the celery juice into the cucumber juice until your body can handle the full celery juice. If it is an actual allergy, please discontinue using celery juice and switch to cucumber juice or another juice that will work for you.

Psoralens

This is a compound found in all fruits and vegetables, and while people say they make your skin sensitive to light, there is no scientific or medical proof. Many medications people take have the warning that they can make them susceptible to the sun. Psoralen is good for you and is what helps to treat skin issues such as eczema and psoriasis.

Pesticides

Inorganic celery makes the list of top ten vegetables with the most residual pesticides. One way to prevent getting celery that is not full of residual pesticides you can purchase organic celery. If you can not find organic celery, you can get pesticides off your celery here in a few ways.

1. Wash it in saltwater - soaking celery in a 10% salt water solution for 20 minutes will get rid of most of the pesticides
2. Soaking it in vinegar will also remove leftover residue from the Celery. You want to use four parts water to 1 part vinegar for 20 minutes. Or you can use full-strength vinegar - whichever one you prefer will work well
3. Clean it with baking soda and water - 1oz baking soda to 100oz of water. Soak for 12-15 minutes.
4. Just rinse it in cold water; this can reduce a lot of the pesticide

Salt content

30mg of sodium in 1 medium stalk - may increase blood pressure and cause fluid retention. We talked about this previously in the book sodium in celery is not the same as the sodium found in sea salt or even table salt. The sodium found in celery is salt clusters that break apart the harmful salt found in packaged food and organic foods.

Oxalates

This molecule is terrible for your health - oxalates are a naturally occurring molecule found in most plants and humans. Too much of this can lead to kidney stones. In plants oxalate helps to get rid of extra calcium by binding to it. Oxalates can be unhealthy if you consume too much of them like most healthy things can be harmful when done to excess.

Sugar

There is sugar in celery juice. Not all sugars are the same. Almost everything you eat has natural or refined sugars. Celery has a very low sugar content. An 8oz glass of celery juice only contains 5 grams of raw sugar. Unlike sodas and other sugar-filled drinks, it is a healthier choice. One of the main differences between natural sugars and added sugars is that natural sugar occurs naturally in foods with health benefits. Added sugars are added during the processing of packaged food and do not provide any health benefits.

Goitrogens

Goitrogens are compounds that are made of sugar and sulfate. These compounds can have undesirable effects on the thyroid and inhibit its iodine uptake. The adverse effects are an unfounded fear and have been significantly exaggerated. - while this compound is found in many vegetables, herbs, and fruits, celery is not. In reading further about Goitrogens, you will find out that it only accounts for 4% of goiter incidences or thyroid issues of the world's population.

Coumarins

Coumarins in celery are toxic to the body - coumarin is a compound found in a variety of foods. It has a sweet fragrant smell and flavor. It is also an ingredient in anticoagulant medications that promote blood circulation, preventing blood clots in your body. There is no way to know just how much coumarin is in any fruit or vegetable. It varies from field to field, state to state, and different areas of the world— the health benefits. Everything in celery juice acts together to offer immune support.

With all the rumors and confusion about celery juice, it is easy to understand why you wouldn't know what to believe. There is so much limited knowledge it's hard to know the facts of what celery juice does and doesn't do. In the next chapter, I have made a list of the most common misconceptions to provide you with the facts instead of rumors.

❧ 4 ❧
BUSTING MYTHS AND MISCONCEPTIONS
DISPELLING COMMON MYTHS

Celery juice doesn't detox your body, the detoxification process starts with the first drink of celery juice. The antioxidants that kill cancer cells immediately leap into action. It heads to your gut, working to restore hydrochloric acid, which aids in digestion; it raises the healthy stomach acid needed to break down foods and proteins. The unique compounds start working to help lower your cholesterol levels. The natural anti-inflammatory polyacetylene starts reducing chronic joint pain, gout, and arthritis. Then it starts working, helping to lower your blood pressure. Two of the most critical detoxification processes are getting the fat deposits, chemicals, and toxins out by producing health enzymes. The enzymes help digestion by flushing toxins out of your digestive tract, which increases circulation in the intestines, which helps with constipation, bloating, puffiness, and gas. This is how celery juice detoxes your body.

The Diuretic effect

Diuretics are medications used as a way to treat high blood pressure or excess water retention. Celery has a trace amount of diuretic in it. One of the benefits of celery juice is to flush out toxins. Sodium salt clusters bind with trace minerals cause the toxins to be flushed out through urination and bowel movements. While researching herb and plant diuretics, I found three of the most common ones: hawthorn, green and black tea, and parsley.

Celery Stalks Health Benefits

Celery stalks do have a lot of health benefits. The most significant difference is that the juicing process removes the fiber. The removal of the fiber makes the juice easier to digest. One of the benefits of drinking celery juice is that it is anti-inflammatory. It starves off the pathogen, flushes out and breaks down viruses, balances your pH, and restores and detoxes your digestive tract. Another benefit of drinking the juice instead of eating celery is it is a good source of vitamin k, folate, and potassium. It is much easier to drink the juice instead of eating an entire bunch of celery.

You Do Not Need to Drink Celery Juice on an Empty Stomach

One of the best benefits of celery juice is it detoxes your liver. When you drink it on an empty stomach, it allows the liver to start healing instead of breaking down a meal's carbs. If you like, you can drink water or water with lemon before having celery juice. Wait 15-20 minutes before drinking your juice.

The Juice May interact with Blood Thinners Due to Vitamin K

Vitamin K can interact with warfarin; it is recommended to take roughly the same amount daily. Like any kind of new health plan or exercise, talk to your doctor.

There is no science behind the celery juice movement

There is a lot of science that does not know about celery. It has been understudied for years. Science still has not learned about the difference between table salt and the type of salt found in celery. Celery has crystallized salt that breaks down table salt and rids it from the body. They know that the vitamins and minerals in the celery juice are healthy and help to rid the body of toxins. The hydrating content helps with many digestive system issues, improves skin, and flushes the body.

Kidney Issues

Celery juice is one of the top ten juices for the bladder and kidneys. Celery is known to remove toxins and contaminants from your kidneys. Celery juice helps to protect from kidney disease. It is also high in vitamins C, B, A, and iron, which help kidney function.

Celery Juice has Nitrates and Nitrites

Nitrates and nitrites are two different types of compounds. Both of these compounds are stable and do not cause harm.

There is confusion between the nitrates found as additives in food products and those that occur naturally. The ones that occur naturally, like in celery, lowers blood pressure and make exercising more effective.

Drinking Celery Juice is Not a Cure-all

No, it isn't a Cure all, nothing is. If you do not eat right, sleep well, and work to have a healthy lifestyle. Juice does heal; you can't expect overnight results. Eating fresh real food and staying away from over-processed packaged foods improves the celery juices' beneficial effects.

5

SHOULD I ADD OTHER INGREDIENTS TO MY JUICE?
ADDING OTHER FOODS, POWDERS, OR INGREDIENTS INTO THE JUICE

Adding other foods, powders, or ingredients into the juice Is not recommended. It dilutes the juice, and you take away from the benefits. The list below all have gifts, just not added with your celery juice. Celery juice, in its purest form, has the most benefits for you. Some things that people suggest adding to the juice are the opposite of what you're trying to accomplish.

Apple Cider Vinegar

While it is alright for you, if you put Apple cider vinegar it in your celery juice, it will ruin its benefits. One of the benefits of celery juice is that it breaks down the acid in your body and flushes it from your system. Adding something high in acid to your juice would defeat the purpose.

Apples

While adding apples to your celery juice to sweeten it up may sound like a good idea, but it will dilute the healing benefits. The apple will keep the salt clusters from breaking down.

Ice

Adding ice to celery juice might make it cooler and dilute the strong flavor of the juice. But it will thoroughly cut any benefits that are in the juice, and it will be useless. It's important to note that water and celery juice are very different.

Lemon Juice

While lemon juice is great with water, do not drink it with celery juice. It dilutes the healing properties.

Fruit

Yes, fruit is an essential part of your daily diet. Just not with your celery juice. If you want fruit, have it in your afternoon smoothie or a late-night snack, Any fruit added to celery juice will ruin the effectiveness.

Greens

Similar to adding vegetables to your celery juice, adding greens have a similar effect. It will hinder the production of natural electrolytes that celery juice promotes. It also causes the brain to work harder to get the same benefits.

Vegetable Juice

Vegetable juices are great to drink, and juices are beneficial. Vegetable juice added to the celery juice will cause your liver to work harder, which negates a detox's purpose. If you are going to add vegetables or vegetable juices, add them to the smoothie you drink later in the day or to another juice.

Collagen

Collagen has many incredible benefits; if you're looking to tone up and feel better, this is a great addition. If you use it with your celery juice, it will put too much bacteria into your gut, causing bloating and constipation. If you are going to use collagen supplements, do not add them to your celery juice. Drinking celery juice gives you a substantial immune boost. Taking collagen powder does the same again. If you use celery juice and collagen supplements, it will overload your immune system, and too much good at one time can be unhealthy.

Protein Powder

Too much protein is harmful to your kidneys. This does not mean that it is terrible for you. Protein helps you gain muscle when you're not overdoing it. One of celery juice's main benefits is detoxing your kidneys.

Activated Charcoal

There are medical conditions that can be aggravated by using charcoal. Dehydration is one of the side effects and is the opposite of what you're trying to do with celery juice. It also is not suitable for those that have constipation or slow digestion. These are both conditions that celery juice improves. Why add something to your juice that does the opposite of what you are achieving.

Fiber

Why not just eat the celery or blend it into a smoothie. Celery is an herb, and the juice is a tonic. Typically when using an herb, you don't use the whole thing. In removing the fiber, you are getting more of the celery's nutrients since it is easier to digest. You aren't missing the fiber from the celery when juiced. You can get it from many other foods and green leafy vegetables.

Leaving in the Pulp

If you leave the pulp in, you mess the natural detoxing properties. You do not have to worry about it being too bland or think if I put this or that in it, It'll be better; That's just not the case. If you do not want to waste the pulp, there are many things you can do with it. Use it for soups; Instead of using cream of celery soup, use the pulp. Make hummus with it and enjoy the added benefits. Another good idea is to make a face mask from it. Celery is so hydrating it would make a great mask.

Using Celery Tablets and Powder

Would you expect to get the same benefits from an orange as you would get from one ground up or make into tablets? It is the same thing with celery power and tables. Using tablets or mixing dried celery in water will not have the same healing benefits as celery juice. Why waste the extra money when you get more help from the juice.

Will my Bowel Movement be Colorful?

No, the only change you may see is a slightly green tint, and that happens if you drink a large quantity of the juice. While you won't experience a difference in color, you will notice a change in frequency. Bowel changes are regular and part of the detox process. If you notice loose stools, it is part of the liver removing toxins and will stop in a few days. If the loose stools and frequent bowel movements are too inconvenient, drink less celery juice and work your way up to the 16oz recommended.

6

HPP AND BOTTLED CELERY JUICE

DRINKING JUICE NOT MADE FROM HOME

When you buy your celery from a juice bar, ask how it is prepared to make sure they are using fresh celery. Oddly enough, Some places add a drop of bleach in the water when washing the celery. That will ruin the benefits and possibly make you sick.

If you are drinking your juice from a bottle, make sure the bottle does not say HPP. HPP stands for high-pressure pasteurization, which means it has been on the shelf that day but was made and delivered by a manufacturing plant. Juices that are made at manufacturing plants are not cold-pressed or fresh. Drinking any liquid that is manufactured has been pasteurized. Pasteurization ruins the secondary compounds and limits the juice's effectiveness. Make sure you check the ingredients in the bottle. If it's pure celery juice, it shouldn't take long to read them. Make sure the first ingredient is celery juice; if not, it doesn't have much liquid.

. . .

Juices from juice bars are seldom freshly squeezed but instead come from concentrates or prepackaged. Usually, the only fresh-squeezed juice comes from oranges. Like the bottled juices, concentrated juices have been pasteurized, have added sugar. The healthy enzymes have been destroyed. The enzymes only come from celery juice that has been freshly juiced.

Another thing to know about juice bars is that their juices have been sweetened with orange, carrot, beet, or apple juice added to it. If you do get your juice from a juice bar, one thing to remember is the added sugar could do more harm than good. Concentrated sugar will feed Candida and overwhelm your endocrine system. Candida is a fungal infection caused by yeast and can cause an infection.

The best way to drink celery juice is freshly made at your home, so you know what is in it.

7

THE LIFESTYLE TO MATCH
MAXIMIZE YOUR BENEFITS WITH THE CORRECT DIET AND LIFESTYLE

Why do you want to cleanse? Do you want it to be a lifestyle or something you occasionally do?

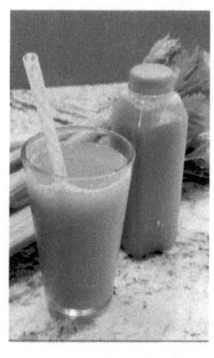

The reason people start a cleanse is to reset their liver. Eating and drinking unhealthy food takes a toll on your body and leads to weight gain. A juice cleanse gives your liver and other organs a chance to flush out toxins and work more effectively. Another reason people juice is to try to change a habit. Maybe you want to start eating healthier, exchange a bag of chips for grapes. A cleanse gives your body a chance to flush out the chemicals you have been eating and start making healthier choices. One of the best ways to get the most out of drinking celery juice is to drink more water. You can drink a glass of water either before or after drinking juice. If you like the taste of lemon, add one to your water for the alkalizing effect and benefit your digestive system. It's important to remember to wait 15-20 minutes between drinking the juice and drinking the water.

Breakfast can be tricky for a few reasons. It's the first meal of the day. We're often in a rush to get out the door and want something quick. When people think of breakfast, they think of eggs, sausage, and toast; there are many other options. Swap out the breakfast filled with fat to a healthier option like oatmeal with some fruit and a morning smoothie. Some people aren't grapefruit fans, but if you are, grapefruits have significant health benefits. Just don't make the mistake of putting sugar on it. Low on time? Grab a banana, an apple or, some people make the overnight oats; these are quick breakfast options.

It's a good idea to limit the number of animal products you eat. Meat is a difficult food to digest, and our bodies need a break. As you age, animal products tend to gather into our lower stomach area, causing that dreaded pouch. During the juicing process, there will be a breakdown of fatty deposits and heavy metals. This breakdown of fat will be eliminated through sweat, urine, and stools. People who eat fewer animal products don't eat as many calories—the amount of fat in your diet decreases, resulting in weight loss.

Dairy is another food you should eat less. Dairy is difficult to digest and is one of the top foods that contribute to clogged arteries. People who are lactose intolerant are not able to fully digest the sugar in dairy. These products can cause loose stools, bloating, and gas for people who have this issue. Lactose intolerance occurs when your small intestine can not properly digest the sugar in daily products.

Eat a well-balanced diet. Most of your calories should come from fresh fruits and vegetables and limited calories from whole grains, lean protein, and nuts. A well-balanced diet is when you eat a variety of food from the food groups mentioned above. While you're juicing, it will expose you to new fruits and vegetables, and maybe you will find some you like.

The good thing with juicing is no matter what diet you are on, juicing works with it. There are many diets people are trying for optimal health. Whether your diet is filled with healthy fats, high protein, high carb, heart-healthy, or plant-based juicing is for you. All foods you eat are going to have some type of a tiring effect on your organs.

People change their diets frequently. There was a time when Slim-Fast was highly popular, then the dinners you could order from dieting companies that would deliver to your home. If you look back on previous diets, it would be interesting to read a list of their ingredients. The diets you hear a lot about now are Keto, interval fasting, and Flexitarian or semi-vegetarian diet, and next year there will probably be new types. With changing diets, your body gets clogged with chemicals, toxins, and heavy metals. Juicing helps to eliminate the toxins in your body while giving you essential vitamins and minerals.

To eliminate temptation while doing a juice cleanse, here are a few suggestions that may help: Make a shopping list - make a list of healthy foods that you like and add many of them. Stick to the plan. When you do not stick to the list, it is easy to look at food and say I'll only eat one. If you have a day where you eat unhealthily, don't be hard on yourself. Eating healthy is a day-by-day process that takes work to become a habit. Get support from friends. Go for a walk with a friend, join a gym, sign up for a yoga class. Suppose you have children, get them up and moving with you. Changing your lifestyle doesn't have to be work; it can be fun too.

Do not stop eating while enjoying your daily juice. Some people have the all-or-nothing approach and use juice as meal replacements. The juice is not a meal replacement. Juicing is something you are doing to ensure you're getting adequate fruits and vegetables. It also helps you get needed nutrients and eliminate buildup in your body. Juicing also adds much-needed vitamins and minerals. If you stop eating regular meals, you probably won't sustain juicing and end up binging on junk food.

If you can limit your alcohol consumption, the benefits of your juice cleanse will last longer. Alcohol is a toxin. If you drink to excess, you will be putting the toxins back into your body, causing your liver to work harder. Alcohol dehydrates the body and puts added stress on the liver to filter this out. With the liver working so hard to eliminate the bad, it's difficult to absorb the good. Alcohol slows down brain tissue growth, and some damage can not be reversed. Cutting out alcohol will make your liver healthier and reduce your chance of developing liver disease.

Limiting or stopping nicotine is essential to your health. Juicing is said to help stop the cycle of addiction. Juicing is great for your heart, lungs, liver and reverses many chronic diseases. Some juices can hope you quit smoking or at least slow down. Some people are under the false belief that smoking calms your nerves. The exact opposite is true. Nicotine can cause anxiety and can exasperate anxiety symptoms. Detoxing and working to heal your body will not have the same effects.

There's a big difference between refined sugar and natural sugar. Natural sugars that occur in fruits and vegetables are essential for good health. Refined sugars have no benefits. Refined sugar increases your risk of high cholesterol, insulin resistance, and blood sugar spikes. Sugar will lower your energy level and raise your risk of having added health concerns. Eating natural sugar has a high level of antioxidants. The nutrients in fruit and vegetables slow down the absorption of sugar.

There are some things you can do in combination with juicing to help you remove toxins. Similar to juicing, sweating is an excellent way to remove toxins from your body. Sweating helps to increase circulation in organs, tissues, and muscles. It also helps to remove excess salt from your system and can help prevent kidney stones. Alcohol and other toxins escape through your skin through sweat.

Sweating is an excellent way to remove toxins. There are many ways to sweat, not just exercise. Native American sweat lodges are not just about having a physical cleanse but a spiritual one. Emotional detoxes are as important as physical ones. There are so many stressors in this day and age: Your job, family, finances, what if your car breaks, and many more. Taking time for yourself is essential to maximize your cleanse.

A sauna is an excellent way to remove toxins from your body. Detoxing in a sauna works hand in hand with your juice detox; they both strengthen your heart and reduce inflammation. Saunas help sore muscles and helps aches and pains. If you are just starting to work out and do yoga the sauna will be beneficial. You can either purchase one or use the one at your local gym.

The Portable Infrared sauna is another choice; You can do right from your home. An infrared sauna works differently than a typical sauna because it heats your body from the inside out. Heating from the inside out helps to accelerate the detox process. This type of sauna also helps with sore muscles, aches and pains. Like celery juice this sauna also helps to clear your skin.

A relatively new way to detox while getting emotional

healing is Chromotherapy. Chromotherapy is also called color lite therapy. Color light therapy is restoring the balance of your body by applying color. These lights are located in an infrared sauna to receive the color lights' full benefits and balance your body.

Dry brushing your skin is another way to get rid of the toxins flushed from your body. Dry brushing involves a daily massage with a dry, stiff-bristled brush. It helps remove dry, flaky skin that occurs during the winter. Other benefits include: increasing circulation, detoxifying, and helping with digestion. Dry brushing is a fast and easy way to increase your juice cleanse benefits, and it doesn't take long.

Earlier I pointed out the benefits of sweating in ways other than exercise and yoga. There are benefits of both of these in addition to detoxing. Increasing flexibility, improving your strength, improved breathing and increased metabolism. There is also a way to relieve stress and help you sleep better at night. When you have had a long busy day at work, I know it's hard to make yourself work out. Even 15 minutes of brisk walking or a nightly yoga routine can help clear your mind and release more toxins through sweat.

There is no way to do all of these daily, and maybe not even weekly; it's a lengthy list. Pick a couple and do one once a day if that's all you can do. The first few that are about nutrition and lifestyle changes are difficult. Again, start slow and work your way to better health. It would be difficult to do those things cold turkey. Make a schedule. Decide the days you are going to work out, and the day you are going to be more productive, and finally, the days you're going to do self-care. On self-care days, do gentle yoga, a hot bath, or a sauna.

Clean out your cupboards and refrigerator, get rid of all of the foods that cause temptation. Replace those foods with fruits, vegetables, and other whole foods. Make sure to get enough proteins, including fish, beans, and vegetables.

Proteins help to fill you up and keep you full for more extended amounts of time. Replace the countertop foods like cake and chips with oranges, apples, or grapes when you want something sweet. I keep cherry tomatoes on my counter along with apples and oranges, for when I feel like grabbing something, I can grab one of those. Stress management is a great way to cut out junk food cravings. When you feel like eating junk, do something healthy, take a walk, do some yoga, or meditate. It has been said that craving will last about 45 seconds; if you can get through that, the worst of it will subside.

Be prepared for some side effects when your body is detoxing. There are toxins in your body that you are removed during your cleanse. These are some types of common toxins that are getting eliminated: heavy metals, pesticides, plastics, industrial chemicals, and bacterial endotoxins. The toxins are removed through your urine, stools, and sweat.

Don't stop juicing if your body has some uncomfortable symptoms when you first start the cleanse. These symptoms are natural, and everyone goes through them. Some common side effects during detox are Headaches, tiredness, and irritability. While juicing is simple to follow, it is a strong medicinal process. These symptoms mean the detox is working, and your body is healing. Your body systems are in chaos while detoxing, and while it works to stabilize itself, you won't always be comfortable. At the start of the juicing process, you are not going to feel great every day. You will have good and bad days. As time goes on, you will start gaining more energy, feeling better, less anxious, and be happier.

Food cravings will happen while you are detoxing from addictive foods like chips and sugar. Include alkaline food in your diet, avoid sugar cravings at meals by eating more protein, and choosing fruits and vegetables. Avoid fried foods by replacing them with healthy alternatives like sweet potatoes, oven-baked zucchini chips, and baked asparagus fries.

While juicing is excellent for your digestive health, you can expect a change in your bowels. At first, your bowels will become more frequent with loose stools. If you were constipated before, you won't be anymore. If you are eating more vegetables than usual, you may experience more gas and bloating than usual. Here are a few more suggestions, eat bitter vegetables and herbs, magnesium supplements, daily physical activity, and eat plenty of non-starchy vegetables.

While going through these changes, do not forget to slow down, relax and reflect on the reason you're doing this. We become focused on what's around us. We forget to stop and feel what's going on in us and our bodies. Throughout your day, pause, notice what's around you, find something that makes you laugh, and always find joy in your day.

Consistency is the key to changing your lifestyle. Establish clear goals and achievable expectations. If you start something, then stop right away, then you don't get the benefits because you quit halfway. If you practice being consistent, it will improve your chances of your effort paying off. Juicing may be something that you have to work at being consistent. After doing it for a while, you will get more used to it, and it will become second nature. If you give up too soon because you don't have enough time or taste good, or for other reasons, you will not know what benefits you did not receive.

It can take anywhere from 18-254 days to start or stop a habit, knowing that helps us realize that changing our lives will take work. It's interesting to note that habit breaking and habit formation are linked in our brains; if you want to quit an unhealthy habit such as eating chips, you need to start a healthy practice like eating an apple. Your motivation matters. What is the reason you want to change the habit? If it's not a reason that is important to you, then it will not stick.

All of the suggestions listed above are just that; suggestions. They are not rules or things you must do to benefit from a cleanse. If you can't do them all, that's understandable, don't beat yourself up. If you can do a few of them, then that's great. You may also backtrack, and that's okay. You can't fail; it's a learning process and a choice.

❧ I ❦
THE SEVEN STEP CLEASING FORMULA

A Seven-Step Plan on How to Execute the Celery Juice Cleanse

During a cleanse, you are going to need a lot of willpower. It is so easy to give in to the temptation to snack on something unhealthy. Once you give in to temptation, it may cause you to be hard on yourself, forgetting to be kind when making mistakes. Starting a juice cleanse is going to cause you stress, especially if it is something new. One way to help minimize the stress making a plan.

I have created a 7 step plan for you to help you start the juicing process and identify the benefits you want to gain from it. When you finish the day and are able to avoid temptation, allow yourself to feel proud. That is amazing you did it. Avoid high-stress situations as best you can. Some people, when stressed, tend to self-soothe with food. Having a well-developed plan will limit some stress, making the cleanse more manageable and more enjoyable.

Stress causes complications within the adrenal glands causing damaged tissues. If you are under constant stress, it triggers fight or flight responses and puts your body under strain. According to medical research, high or continuous pressure increases your chance of heart disease. Through reading this book, we have learned that juicing can reverse the effects of stress and what it does to the body.

❋ 1 ❋
STEP 1: DECIDE WHEN TO START YOUR CLEANSE
WHY ARE YOU MAKING THE CHOICE TO CLEANSE?

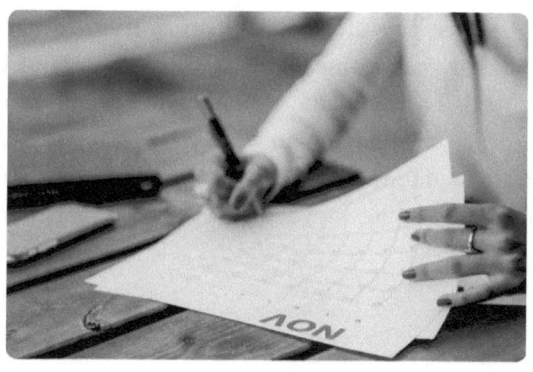

Normally, people decide to cleanse for liver health. Overeating junk keeps your body from functioning correctly and efficiently. Your body is getting to rest during a cleanse because it isn't working hard to digest foods. Is this enough of a reason for you to start drinking celery juice daily? Do you need more reasons to start the cleanse?

Do you wake up sluggish, sometimes it is almost like you woke up more tired than you felt when you went to sleep? If there is no medical reason for what you are experiencing, I will look at my daily habits. Are you working at a desk all day long without much physical activity? Are you going home, grabbing a quick unhealthy dinner, sitting on the couch watching television until you go to bed? If you answer yes to these questions, you might want to do a celery juice cleanse.

Lose some weight? If you want to lose weight, juicing is your best friend. You don't have to follow a lot of rules; there are not strict regiments. You simply add more nutrients to your body that you don't normally eat. Instead of eating at a restaurant or grabbing a burger, you can make a delicious and healthy juice. If you tend to snack during the day or while relaxing while watching TV grab some juice instead.

Do you have stomach issues? Do you suffer from a slow digestive system, do you feel sick the day after eating something unhealthy, or suffer from bloating after eating? Eating fatty foods for years causes your digestive system to become overwhelmed. The nutrients contained in juice make it easier to be absorbed. Depending on what you eat, it can take up to three hours to digest. Imagine how you and your body feels with the food setting in your stomach for that amount of time.

STEP 2: LIMIT CAFFEINE
CAFFEINE IS NOT YOUR FRIEND

Caffeine is not your friend. Caffeine makes it challenging to fall asleep, and sleep is vital for your body. Your body needs to rest so the juice can do its job. And caffeine increases stress hormones, and you need to avoid that during a cleanse. It causes these things by increasing your cortisol and adrenaline levels which increases energy. Caffeine slightly increases pH levels which can cause gastric ulcers, acid reflux, and irritable bowel syndrome.

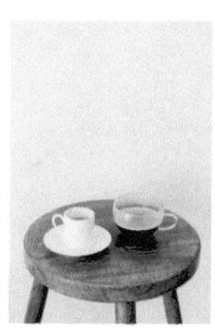

Start eliminating the primary sources of caffeine. Chocolate is a source of caffeine that many people do not realize. Energy drinks, if you think coffee has caffeine, energy drinks have so much more. Plus, energy drinks can have serious health effects, especially on children, teenagers, and young adults—caffeinated teas, like green tea and black tea. While tea has many benefits to your health, as stated earlier, caffeine has many effects that are not beneficial. Pop is loaded with caffeine, unhealthy sugars and is hard on your kidneys. Decaf coffee, while decaf coffee doesn't have as much caffeine as regular coffee, depending on where it's sourced, it may have anywhere from 0.1%-3%.

You do not have to stop caffeine suddenly; in fact, quite the opposite. I would suggest slowly cutting down. If you have ever tried quitting caffeine cold turkey, you know the severe symptoms of withdrawing. If you use multiple caffeine sources like pop and energy drinks, start sipping your pop instead of downing it. Drink half of the energy drink, half a cup of coffee. You usually want to start weaning off of caffeine the week before you begin juicing. Don't forget the water, as your body is while coming off your caffeine dependency.

A primary reason to give up caffeine during a cleanse is the purpose of cleansing is to get a break from your daily diet. Caffeine is a diuretic, and it can interfere with the natural cleanse you are trying to do while you are doing the juice cleanse. Removing toxins from caffeine causes your liver to work harder. Caffeine is one of the main things you want to avoid while cleansing.

STEP 3: ELIMINATE PROCESSED FOOD
ONE OF THE BEST THINGS YOU CAN DO FOR YOUR HEALTH

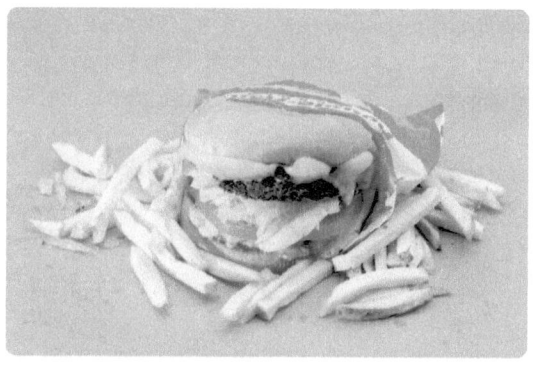

What are processed foods? These are foods that have been altered to be more filling, last longer, and taste better. Processed foods increase your risk of cancer because of the large amounts of chemicals in them. These foods digest quickly, meaning it does not take much energy or many calories. They contain a lot of sugar which makes sense since they're very addicting. Since they are so high in calories, it is easy to overeat them and not even realize it. Many of the ingredients in processed foods are banned in other countries because of the chemicals they contain. It's scary to think that some common foods we eat aren't even allowed in other countries because they are unhealthy.

One of the best things you can do for your health is to eliminate processed foods. You are going to start juicing. Your goals are to detox and feel great. Then you look at that box of macaroni and cheese thinking, should I? One package won't hurt, right? Yes, yes, it will. Processed food has little if no health benefits. If you look at the ingredients, there are many of them, and most you can't even pronounce.

Eliminating processed foods helps to improve your health. It improves your brain and your mood. It improves your brain health because processed foods are filled with fat, which causes memory loss and difficulty learning. Foods that are processed have also been shown to worsen symptoms of mood disorders. When you cut out those types of foods, it will also improve your looks. The inflammatory properties cause acne and aggravate skin conditions. It is not easy to cut these foods out of your diet. They are quick and easy to make and packaged in appealing bags or boxes.

4

STEP 4: LIMIT FATS
FATS ARE HARD FOR YOUR BODY TO BREAK DOWN

Fats are one of the most challenging foods for your liver to break down. The deposits are highly absorbable, and they grab toxins and store them in your body. Because of how absorbent they are, they act as fuel for many viruses. In juicing, it helps break down the fat for the liver and then eliminate it. Not all fat is bad, and we do need fat in our diets. Healthy fat helps us to absorb specific vitamins that are essential for health. Any fat unused by your body's cells convert into body fat.

Bloating is one symptom of eating products high in fat. The way that fat affects our brain is they get into the bloodstream, slowing down blood flow to the brain. Fats affect your cholesterol levels, causing them to rise. It can also just make you feel gross.

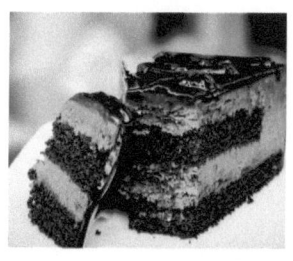

The juicing process eliminates the fatty deposits from your diet, decreasing your cholesterol levels, improving brain function, and helps you feel better.

Too much fat in your diet contributes to high cholesterol, increasing your risk of heart disease, strokes, and diabetes. Small amounts of fat can harm your health. A small number of fat calories can raise your risk of heart disease by 23%. Even healthy fats can cause health concerns, causing fat deposits to cause plaque to form in your arteries. Both good and bad fat can cause you to gain weight, which increases your risk of diabetes.

If you're overeating fat, it will give you bad breath, and you will need to use mouthwash and brush your teeth more often during the day. As stated many times, it will cause stomach issues, especially if you do not include many vegetables in your diet. All around, you just won't feel right. Fat causes inflammation, and that makes people feel sluggish and tired.

STEP 5: DRINK MORE WATER
WATER IS THE MOST IMPORTANT NUTIRENT

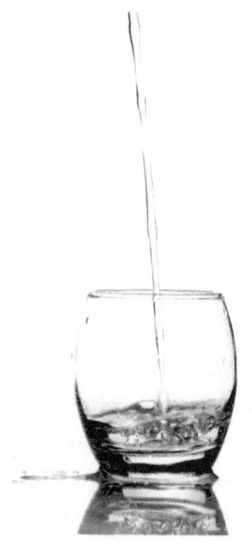

Water has many of the same benefits as doing a juice cleanse. It helps to get rid of waste through sweating, urinating, and stools. It assists the digestion process by helping your body break down food and absorb its nutrients.

You can improve your mood when you stay hydrated and help your skin look healthy.

Water is an essential part of your daily life. You can't function without it. It supports the elimination of wastes and makes sure your joints have enough lubrication. It brings moisture to all tissues and organs and helps to digest food. We are continually losing water during the day through sweat, urine, and bowel movements. Juicing creates a partnership between the juice and the water causing hydration to last longer. Knowing this does not mean you do not have to slow down drinking water; just the opposite is true. The majority of your body is made up of water, making it essential to keep it working correctly.

Do you get tired during the day, drink a glass of water. Having trouble concentrating, drink a glass of water. It also helps you to control your weight because thirst can be confused with hunger. When I feel hungry at an odd time of day, I will generally drink some water, wait about 10 minutes and see if the craving goes away. If it does, I know I was thirsty and not hungry.

Experts say during a juice cleanse to drink half your weight in ounces of water. Other things that should help determine the amount of water you should consume are: Where do you live? If you live in a warm, dry state, it makes sense that you'll lose more water than someone who lives in a cooler state. What are your daily habits? Are you someone who does a lot of sitting or exercise all day? If you are an active person, you will want to drink more water.

Drinking water when you first wake up gives your organs some lubricant and helps wake up your liver. It also helps your body to flush out toxins and allows your brain to work better. If your brain doesn't get the hydration it needs, it will cause you to feel drained. If your goal is to lose weight, water will get your metabolism up and running.

You may wonder why you should juice cleanse when it seems like water does the same thing. While water does do many of the same things, there are benefits of juicing that water does not provide. Juicing helps your body to recover and detox on a larger scale quicker than drinking water. Water doesn't give you calories which could cause you to lose too many calories during the day, and you may feel drained. Juicing does provide you with calories helping to not get that drained feeling. During juicing, your immune system gets a boost with all of the additional vitamins your body is getting.

❧ 6 ☙

STEP 6: LISTEN TO YOUR BODY
HOW AM I FEELING RIGHT NOW?

Learning to listen to your body may be a new experience for you. At first, it is hard to do, so often we go through life thinking we need to ignore our bodies and do what we are "supposed to." While growing up, your parents told you to clean your plate and receive a lecture if you didn't.

Some people get confused at the notion of listening to themselves. They do not realize a difference between your brain telling your body it craves something and listening to your body. How do you feel when you eat pie versus when you have an apple or salad.

When you start listening to your body, your brain may trick you. Brains learn what chemicals are released when you eat a particular food, and it wants to keep those chemicals coming. If you eat chocolate knowing that it releases serotonin which is a chemical that makes you feel good, it may help you understand why you're experiencing the craving. Knowing this may help you get through the urge, or you can see if a healthy food can cause a similar feeling.

THE CELERY JUICE CLEANSE HACK: A 7 STEP GUIDE TO F...

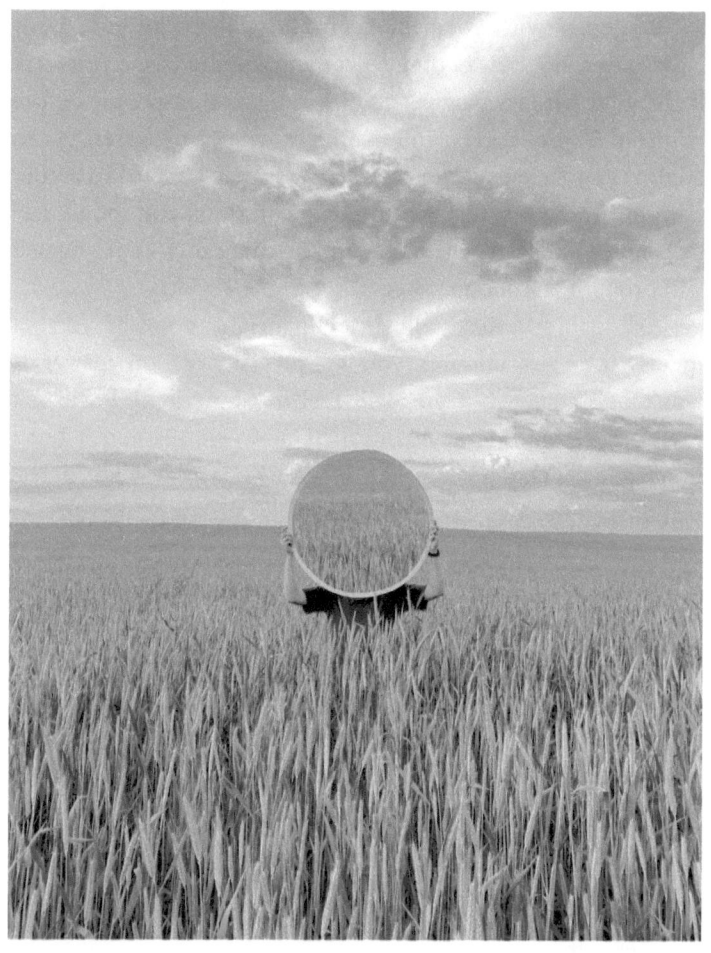

Be gentle with yourself. Learning to listen to your body isn't something that's going to come naturally. Since you were little, your parents taught you to listen to other people before yourself. There is a fear in learning to listen to yourself. As an adult if you have experienced trauma it may be hard to reconcile your thoughts, feelings and how you think you should feel or think. Listening to yourself and learning to accept yourself will probably be a long process.

Ask yourself, how am I feeling right now? If you sit quietly for a few minutes, you will probably get an answer. It won't be audible, but you will feel it. Sometimes I will ask myself if I could do anything right now, what would it be? I don't get a crazy answer like travel the world; I get a real response. One day asking myself this question, my answer was dance. I got up, put on some music, and danced, and it felt great. That is hard to remember to do.

Movement is a great way to get to know your body. Get up early, do yoga, take a walk, do something that causes you to get out of your head. Moving is a great way to connect to your body, and it brings you into the present moment. Another tool I use is meditation, one of the best ways to learn to listen to yourself.

STEP 7: CHOOSE THE CORRECT FOODS
WHAT YOU SHOULD EAT

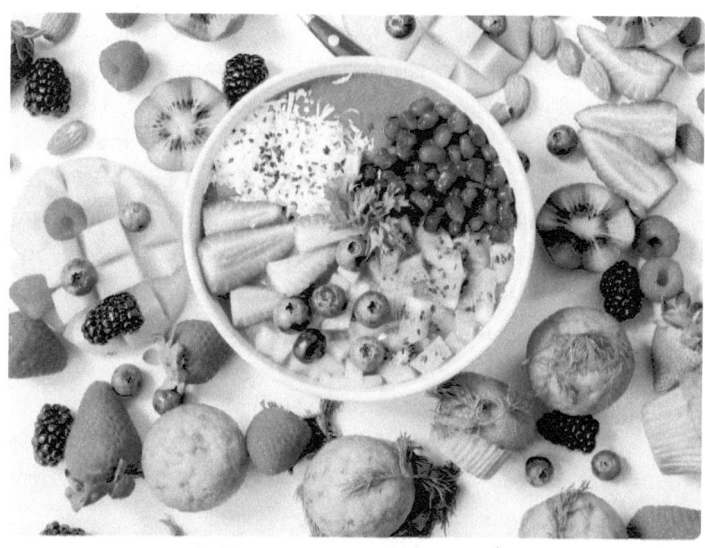

Now that you know what not to eat, let's focus on what to eat. Starting on a juice cleanse does not mean the night before you should eat a huge, sugar-filled meal willed with fats. You should do the exact opposite. Your juice cleanse will be so much more challenging if you don't prepare yourself for it by eating healthy. People will often use juicing to go back and forth between eating healthy, then going back to their old way of eating, and then starting another juice cleanse. Using cleanses and detoxes can become as addictive as using laxatives or diuretics as a way to undo the adverse effects of overeating; if you're someone that tends to do this, look into your relationship with food.

If you start changing the way you eat before starting the cleanse, you will have better results. Start eating more vegetables, fruits, nuts, and seeds, and healthy protein. Eat simple small meals that are easy to digest and are full of green leafy vegetables. If you crave soups, there are many non-creamy grain-free ones you can make. About five days after starting the juice cleanse, cravings for unhealthy foods begin to fade. Once you start eating better, you will be able to figure out when you're hungry and eat enough. You start wanting to eat healthily, and you crave the taste of fresh foods.

Add color to your plate. Not only does color make your food look more appetizing, but you will also get more vitamins and minerals. Eat a variety of salad greens. When you shop for salad greens, get a variety of greens. Look for your favorite greens and some you haven't tried before just to see what you think. There are some sweet fruits and vegetables to satisfy a craving. A few examples of sweeter vegetables are green peppers, sweet potatoes, and squash. Most importantly, don't let eating become boring, have fun, blend different flavors just to see how it tastes. If you don't already, you may just learn to love cooking.

When you start focusing on having a healthy diet, you will start cooking at home more, eating breakfast daily, and taking your lunch to work. Since you are no longer eating processed food, you now prepare your lunch before work. Like cooking at home, bringing your lunch to work is a twofold benefit.

You not only are eating better, but you're also saving money too.

Eat dinner by 7:00 pm. After dinner, you can have some raw nuts or a smoothie to help appease your hunger. Nutritionists have typically recommended having three meals a day with 2-3 snacks. Take your time while eating, make a conscious effort to pay attention to how the food tastes. It takes time for your brain to realize when you're feeling full. Never think of any food as being off-limits. When you do that, you start thinking of it more often, which may cause you to binge on them.

If you have a sluggish digestive system, you may want to start eating steamed or baked vegetables before working up to raw ones. Years of eating unhealthy foods take a toll on your digestive system. During a juice cleanse, you will be getting the enzymes you're missing, and you will notice the change in how you feel.

8
HOW TO MAKE THIS A HABIT THAT WILL CHANGE YOUR LIFE
PLAN AND EXECUTE

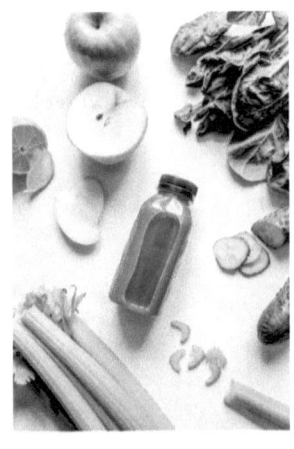

Juicing can be the first step in making healthier choices. When you're finished with your 30 day cleanse, you will feel amazing. You will want to continue feeling this way. Feeling good each day is possible! You can make all of the same choices and keep juicing. You have discovered many of the benefits of juicing. Why stop now. Make it a part of your daily life. Each morning make yourself a juice, just like you have been. Now, instead of just celery juice, you can start experimenting. Ask yourself the question of what benefit do you want to get from juicing. Do you want added energy? Look for a recipe that says for added energy. If you have gone to the store and read the ingredients, some combine many different juices. Seeing all the different combinations can cause you to feel overwhelmed. That's why you want to find a book or search the internet for beginner juice recipes. Beginner juice recipes will have fewer ingredients and will give you a chance to work your way up to juices with more ingredients. Beginner juicing tips can help you find the type of juicer you want or if you want a juicer. Some people use a blender and strain out the whole parts. What benefits you get from juicing are endless.

During the juice, you gave up caffeine. You've made it through the withdrawal and detox process. You can choose if you want to start consuming caffeine again or not. If you did a 30 day cleanse and gave it up for the entire time, you might want to start slowly. During this time, you have probably become more sensitive to caffeine's effects, so introduce it gradually. Don't jump right back into drinking a full cup of coffee or a glass of pop all at once. Consuming caffeine suddenly may have an adverse effect on you. If you can, try to limit the amount of alcohol you drink and don't drink any for the first week after your cleanse. Your liver enjoyed the break from working so hard let it get used to breaking down and digesting food slowly. If you can help it, do not go back to eating high sugar and processed foods. Going back to old habits will start the process of your body working hard and your liver becoming sluggish all over again.

Watch the amounts of fat and protein you're eating. When you eat fats, make sure they are healthy versus unhealthy fats. By now, you have learned the difference; use your knowledge. Make sure you're eating high-quality, skinless protein if you are eating animal products. Starting to consume dairy suddenly may have adverse effects as well.

Dairy has a tendency to cause constipation, so make sure to keep eating high fiber. While on the cleanse, you started listening to your body's needs and listening to yourself. Continuing to eat whole foods instead of junk food will help to keep you self-aware. While doing your juice cleanse, your skin started to look great. If you continue eating healthy, your skin will continue to look healthy. Be careful of sugars. It is easy for them to sneak back into your diet. Many drinks or juices that claim to be natural aren't natural. If you read the label, you may find ingredients that show their added sugars and other ingredients. Instead of drinks with added sugars, you can drink water with lemon or drink water with mint and cucumber. There are also caffeine-free and herbal fruit teas that are great options.

Don't forget to hydrate. Continue drinking enough water daily to help aid your digestion. You've been getting a lot of extra hydration during your juice cleanse, so try to decrease the hydration slowly. Continue to eat your fruits and vegetables. You have gone through the hard work of making them essential to your diet. You know firsthand the benefits. Try to aim for five servings of vegetables daily and two servings of fruit. During your cleansing, you have started exercising and exploring different ways to sweat. Keep this habit. Sweating will help you to continue to detox and flush out toxins. Keep moving! Exercising, doing yoga, walking, or stretching are all ways to continue moving. Not only does it make you healthy, but it also makes you feel great too.

Finding whole foods can be less convenient than grabbing frozen or canned foods, but the health benefits are enormous. During the cleanse, you have learned so much about the difference between whole food and processed foods. Whole Foods are full of healthy nutrients that we need to be healthy. They have raw sugar instead of processed sugar. Knowing this is important because your body is better able to process natural sugar. Whole Foods are heart-healthy. They're packed with antioxidants and rich in nutrients. Whole Foods are high in fiber, supporting a healthy digestive system and helping you feel full longer. The higher fiber content helps to keep your gut healthy because it is rich in prebiotics.

Whole Foods do cost more, and if you do not have a lot

of money, this can make it hard. Do the best you can. Any improvement is a win. It can make preparing food time-consuming because you will need to plan and prepare your meals. It can lead to stress if you feel you can only eat whole foods. It is essential to remember you're doing the best you can and continue to go easy on yourself. One way to help with time is to plan and prepare your meals weekly or daily. It doesn't need to be complicated. What ingredients do you already have? Make use of the fruits and vegetables to save time having to go out shopping—layout what you will eat all week on Sunday Afternoon. Plan your meals, including snacks, and if you're going to have a healthy dessert like fruit salad, make it earlier in the week. If you don't want to do it once a week, do it for a few days in advance. Make sure the food you are preparing food you enjoy so you look forward to eating it. Enjoying what you eat is essential to your diet; if you do not want to eat your food, why bother sticking with your new plan.

If you can't or don't want to continue eating whole foods, the next best thing is learning to read food labels. Please don't believe what it says on the front of the box. Marketing companies make a lot of claims that aren't true. Always read the nutrition label and ingredient list. Always check the serving size; if a bag of frozen vegetables contains eight servings and the serving size 1/4 cup, there's a good chance it's not going to fill you up. Calories per serving are essential to read to determine your calories accurately. Check the amount of sodium that is in the food. What type of fats are in the food, no saturated fats, no hydrogenated fats. All fat can damage your heart. If you're getting grain products, make sure it is a whole grain. Reading a food label is confusing and hard to learn how to do correctly. There are so many phone apps out there now that you can probably find one that can help out.

Continue to journal. Food journaling is excellent for

mindful eating. You will be keeping track of what you eat and the number of calories you are getting. Many times by the end of the day, you have forgotten what you ate earlier in the day. Journaling is a way to prevent this from happening. It also helps you to know the times of day you get the most hungry. You will discover if you are eating out of boredom or if you are an emotional eater. If you are eating out of boredom, you can find ways to distract yourself and do something healthy. Go for a walk, listen to music or get up and move. If you're an emotional eater, you can take steps to learn your triggers. If stress is a trigger, find what helps you to release tension. If being upset is a trigger for you finding ways you can find a way to feel better than with food. Learning to soothe yourself is a tool that is always needed.

Some people feel better after a nice warm bath, doing yoga, exercising, or painting. Find what works for you. You can Keep your journaling short. It doesn't have to be pages. A helpful benefit about journaling is you will find out if you have a food sensitivity and what food makes you feel better or bothers you. Food journaling can help you find out how you are eating, affecting what and how you eat. You will learn your real eating habits. Are you eating as much healthy food as you think you are? Are you trying to trick yourself into believing you are doing better than you are? These are some of the answers you will find when you keep a journal.

AFTERWORD

Thank you for making it through to the end of *The Celery Juice Cleanse Hack*, let's hope it was informative and able to provide you with all of the tools you need to achieve your goals whatever they may be.

There is so much confusion over what the celery juice cleanse is that it's hard to decide fact from fiction. You will find out what a juice cleanse is and how it will benefit you and your body. Your body and mind are connected to the food you eat, and juicing can improve both. When your digestive system is not functioning well, you don't feel well, and it will have a negative impact on your moods. Celery juice is a great way to detox your body from all of the chemicals you consume in your daily life. If this is your first cleanse, you will learn what to expect when you begin juicing: what you should add, if anything, to your juice. You will learn about detox symptoms, how to make them less harsh, and the best ways to deal with them. A step-by-step guide will help you move through the juicing process with ease and prepare for the cleanse. You will discover if juicing is part of a lifestyle you want to keep or if you're going to use it as the occasional pick-me-up. If you're going to make it part of your lifestyle, there are suggestions on how you can do that. We will explore common myths and misconceptions about what exactly celery does and does not do. How you can incorporate juicing in your daily life and why you would want to. By the end of the book, we will help you answer whether celery juice has the benefits people claim.

www.ingramcontent.com/pod-product-compliance
Lightning Source LLC
Chambersburg PA
CBHW021441070526
44577CB00002B/245